Praise for

Driving Mr. Yogi

"Baseball at its best is a game of relationships — fathers and sons, mothers and daughters, veterans and rookies. In *Driving Mr. Yogi,* one of America's finest sportswriters writes about the magical relationship between two of the greatest Yankees ever, Yogi Berra and Ron Guidry, a great catcher and a great pitcher from different times. Any baseball fan would love to be at spring training, sun shining, smell of mowed grass in the air, and just listen to the stories of those two wonderful men. Harvey Araton lets us do just that."

— **Joe Posnanski, author of *The Machine* and *The Soul of Baseball***

"Harkens back to an era when ballplayers were teammates because of the uniform they wore, not the games they played. *Driving Mr. Yogi* is as sweet as the unlikely friendship between Berra and his designated chauffeur Ron 'Gator' Guidry who, along with author Harvey Araton, handles this precious baseball cargo with requisite TLC."

— **Jane Leavy, bestselling author of *The Last Boy* and *Sandy Koufax***

"Spending time with Yogi Berra, and experiencing his wit, wisdom, and wonder, is a unique pleasure, as Ron Guidry, a special guy himself, can attest. Now thanks to Harvey Araton's delightful book you, too, can get to know one of the world's great treasures as Louisiana Lightning does, through his eyes, and revel in a remarkable relationship between the Hall of Fame catcher and great Yankee pitcher that exists far beyond the ballfield." — **Tim McCarver, sportscaster, FOX Sports**

"Yogi Berra was the hero of my youth. Like Ron Guidry, one of the greatest gifts in my career of being mayor was to become Yogi's friend. He and Ron are unique Americans and in *Driving Mr. Yogi* readers everywhere will come to see just how special their friendship is." — **Rudy Giuliani**

"How would you like to hang out with Yogi Berra and Ron Guidry during spring training? Funny and sweet, *Driving Mr. Yogi* transports you there." — **Jim Bouton, former major league player and author of *Ball Four***

"Hop in, sit back and enjoy the ride with Yogi and Gator. With grace and humor, Harvey Araton makes certain it will put a smile on your face."

— **Tom Verducci, bestselling author (with Joe Torre) of *The Yankee Years***

Driving Mr. Yogi

*Yogi Berra, Ron Guidry, and
Baseball's Greatest Gift*

Harvey Araton

MARINER BOOKS
HOUGHTON MIFFLIN HARCOURT
BOSTON   NEW YORK

To the memory of Gilbert Araton, my father,
and Morris Finkelstein, my uncle, who both took me to see
Yogi Berra and the Yankees play for the first time in 1962.

First Mariner Books edition 2013

www.hmhco.com

Library of Congress Cataloging-in-Publication Data
Araton, Harvey.
Driving Mr. Yogi : Yogi Berra, Ron Guidry, and baseball's greatest gift / Harvey Araton.
p. cm.
ISBN 978-0-547-74672-2 (hardback)   ISBN 978-0-544-00227-2 (pbk.)
1. Berra, Yogi, date. 2. Guidry, Ron, date. 3. Baseball players — United States — Biography.
4. New York Yankees (Baseball team) I. Title.
GV865.B4A78 2012
796.3570922 — dc23
[B]   2011052544

Book design by Brian Moore

Printed in the United States of America
DOC 10 9 8 7 6 5 4 3 2

Contents

Prologue

The one thing Yogi Berra and Ron Guidry have most in common and is obvious to everyone is that they are so unaffected by fame that you have to wonder if they even know that they were great players.

—GOOSE GOSSAGE

Morning in Florida usually put Yogi Berra in the best of moods, but Ron Guidry could see right away that his old friend was cranky, not his usual sprightly self.

Normally Berra would be waiting for Guidry in front of his hotel, smiling and waving at the many well-wishers and fans until his ride to the park pulled up to the curb. But not this day. Not this time. As Guidry approached, Berra was pacing, and Guidry could hear him through the open passenger side window mumbling under his breath: "Goddamn, son of a . . ."

Guidry checked his watch to see if he was late — which was one of the few things that always made Berra grumpy — but, no, he was actually a few minutes early. He leaned across the seat and pushed open the door.

As Berra climbed into the truck, Guidry said, "Yogi, what's the problem?"

"Ah, I just found that I got to fly to LA Friday morning," Berra said.

"LA?" Guidry said. "What the hell for?"

Guidry pulled away from the hotel, out into traffic, on the way to the Yankees' spring training complex.

Berra complained, "I got to make an affliction commercial."

Guidry looked at him with bemusement, thinking, *Is he doing something with some kind of hospital?*

"You know," Berra said, "with that goddamn duck."

And then it struck Guidry what Berra was talking about.

"You mean the Aflac commercial?" he said.

"Yeah," Berra growled, "that damn duck."

Guidry burst out laughing, couldn't stop, to the point where he had to pull over to the side of the road. He sat there for a minute, practically doubled over, reddened face against the wheel.

And then, out of the corner of his eye, he looked over at Berra, who was laughing at himself, suddenly in on his own joke.

Guidry shook his head and thought, *Anytime you can share a laugh like this with this man, it's a great moment.*

1

The Pickup

Ron Guidry steered his white Ford F-150 pickup with the NEW YORK YANKEES plates to the curb of the Continental Airlines arrivals area at Tampa International Airport. He pushed open the driver's side door, stood up, and looked around for the airport traffic attendant. He hoped it would be the same sympathetic fellow he had encountered the previous year.

"Can I help you?" the guy had said when he'd noticed Guidry looking around uneasily.

"Yeah, I'm waiting for a highly valued package," Guidry had replied. "Are you a baseball fan?"

The attendant had said no, not really. But when Guidry had told him who he had come to pick up — "I'm waiting for a little dude by the name of Berra" — he had gotten the thoroughly predictable response.

The attendant's eyes had widened. Of course he had heard of Berra. "Yogi's coming?" he had said. "Why don't you go inside and wait for him? I'll watch your truck."

Unfortunately, a year had passed, and now all Guidry saw was a uniformed female employee who eyed him suspiciously as he edged a few steps from the truck in the direction of the terminal. Guidry decided not to risk it, because the only thing worse than not being where Berra expected him to be would be having the truck towed and having no ride at all.

So Guidry stood like a sentry in his white, short-sleeved, button-down shirt, which hung just below the belt line of his dark slacks. At age sixty, he was starting to turn gray, his combed-back hair barely clinging to its natural dark glint. Otherwise, the man celebrated by Yankees fans as "Louisiana Lightning" remained trim and tanned enough to be mistaken at a glance for a player in his prime.

It was late on the afternoon of February 22, 2011. Being in Tampa at this time of year was a ritual of late winter for Guidry, a foreshadowing of the calendar spring. After his retirement from the Yankees in 1989, he had returned every year as a special camp instructor, with the exception of the two years he had served as the team's pitching coach, 2006 and 2007, and the strike year, 1995, when baseball had tried to ram replacement players down the public's throat during spring training. There was no way he was showing up for that.

He never flew to Tampa, preferring instead to load his truck for the eleven-hour drive from his handsome gated home on about seventy rustic acres outside Lafayette, Louisiana, a straight shot on Interstate 10 across Mississippi, Alabama, and on into northern Florida's western flank. From there, Guidry would head south on Interstate 75, the final leg into the Yankees' training base, directly across Dale Mabry Highway from Raymond James Stadium, home of the NFL's Tampa Bay Buccaneers.

By this breezy Tuesday afternoon, he had already been in camp for about a week, having timed his arrival, as always, to pitchers and catchers. It never took long — a workout or two — for Guidry to get his head back in the game. But his heart beat to a different rhythm, to a conviction that no spring training could really begin until the most famous catcher of all had arrived.

That would be Lawrence Peter Berra, the American icon with the most endearing nickname known to man, bestowed on him by a childhood friend because of the yoga-like position he assumed while

THE PICKUP • 3

waiting for his turn to bat during neighborhood sandlot games on benchless St. Louis ball fields. Guidry was at the airport to pick up the eighty-five-year-old "package," his dear friend — "my best friend," he would say, as a matter of fact — coming for his annual stay of several weeks.

"It's like I'm the valet," Guidry said. "Actually, I *am* the valet."

And when Berra hit town, there could be no excuse for failing to be there on time to meet him. Everyone who knew the old man understood the one essential requirement to maintaining a relationship with him: he did not accept lateness, most of all in himself. Guidry knew it as well as anyone in Berra's immediate family: "Yogi is never late."

So there was little chance, Guidry reasoned, that flight 518 from the notoriously congested Newark Liberty International Airport would dare fail to touch down at its appointed time. Not with Berra — a man who inspired people earthbound and airborne alike to please him — on board.

The punctual side of Yogi Berra was never plainer — and more painful — to those closest to him than the previous summer, after he took a fateful step just outside the front door of his home in Montclair, New Jersey, on a Friday afternoon, July 16, 2010.

It was an emotional time for Berra, reeling from the deaths of the most famous of all Yankees voices, the longtime public-address announcer Bob Sheppard on July 11 and "the Boss" himself, George Steinbrenner, two days later. It was also the day before Old-Timers' Day at Yankee Stadium — the Yankees being the team that originated the concept and the last to continue it, primarily because they continued to churn out players to celebrate, decade after decade. Not that anyone had planned it this way, but the timing of the deaths was another clear illustration that no organization in sports did pomp and pathos quite like the Yankees.

Given the magnitude of the occasion, Berra decided it might be a good idea to tidy up his appearance. He normally had his hair cut at a local barbershop. But out of respect for Old-Timers' Day and the an-nual Hall of Fame induction ceremonies in Cooperstown, New York, eight days later, he made an appointment at the Classic Look, his wife Carmen's favorite salon on Bloomfield Avenue, just across the town border in Verona. In anticipation of having to sign a fair number of autographs, Yogi Berra, metrosexual, whose thick, gnarly fingers had borne the brunt of nineteen years behind the plate, also opted for a manicure.

Checking his watch, anxious to get into his car for the short drive, he forgot about the cracked cement on the front step. He caught his foot and went down fast, face first. Soon blood was everywhere, in a quickly widening pool on the ground, all over his face and clothes.

Having celebrated his eighty-fifth birthday two months earlier, on May 12, he was considered in excellent health for a man his age, but he had been taking the blood thinner Coumadin since being diagnosed with an irregular heartbeat in his seventies.

So here is what Berra, a man of his word and of unalterable rou-tine, chose to do next: he slowly and achingly got up, staggered back inside the house to change his shirt and locate a towel in a largely fu-tile attempt to stanch the bleeding from his nose — which had taken the worst of the fall — and drove himself to the salon with one hand on the wheel.

There Denise Duke, the stylist, was already wondering what the heck was going on. Berra was late, and that had never happened be-fore when he'd had an appointment with her. He was, in fact, usually a half-hour early. But when he arrived, bleeding profusely and looking as white as a ghost, she became nearly hysterical.

An attractive blond in her midforties, Duke had known the Ber-ras for some time, and as a loyal Yankees fan, she loved doting on Yogi, whom she liked to call "my boyfriend," especially when Carmen was around. But in all seriousness, she marveled at how unassuming Berra was for a major celebrity and how well he handled the salon patrons, who could never resist getting into his space and telling him what big fans they were as a prelude to asking for an autograph. He almost never refused.

Once, Duke introduced her nephew—a gangly high school baseball player who happened to be a catcher—to her famous friend. Berra signed the boy's mitt and several weeks later inquired as to how he was doing. Not so well, she said; he had torn up a knee and was going to need it rebuilt.

"He's broken already?" Berra asked.

What did he mean by "broken"? Then she realized this was just Berra-speak—"nothing fancy, plain English," and part of why so many people related to him so well.

Unfortunately, he wasn't relating to her when she begged him to forget about the manicure and get to the hospital immediately. "I'm fine; it'll stop," he said of the bleeding. That didn't seem likely to Duke, who was aware that Berra was on Coumadin—as her father had been—and knew how things could quickly get out of control.

Berra was also breathing heavily and appeared to be trembling. She feared he might be in serious trouble, so she summoned a young police officer who just happened to be standing outside the shop in the small strip mall. He was of no help: Berra charmed the starstruck officer into agreeing with him that he was OK.

While her colleagues tended furiously to Berra's facial cuts, Duke rushed through the manicure and haircut and told him she would drive him home. No, he said, he'd drive himself home, and besides, she couldn't possibly drive his car.

"What are you saying, that I can't drive a Jaguar?" she said.

That's right, he insisted; only he could drive the Jaguar. But he offered her a compromise: she could ride with him, if that would make her happy.

Anxious to get him home however she could, where hopefully Carmen could talk some sense into him, Duke agreed to the terms. She asked her shampoo girl to follow them so that she would have a ride back to the shop, but she regretted this arrangement as soon as

Berra pulled onto Bloomfield Avenue, a crowded roadway, and began drifting from one lane to the other.

"Yogi, be careful," she said.

"It's OK," he said, assuring her that other cars always had a habit of avoiding his.

How, exactly, was that? she asked skeptically. He shrugged. That apparently was just how it was.

When they reached Berra's quiet street, Duke asked if Carmen was at home. He said he didn't know. Then the bleeding octogenarian with a crimson paper towel stuck to his nose turned to her and snapped, "I hope she isn't, because if she sees me bringing *you* home with me, you'll be bleeding worse than me."

Under the circumstances, Duke didn't know whether to crack up or cry. But when she saw the bloodstains on the front walk, she began to believe that this most unusual man must indeed have an angel guiding him.

It was an absolute miracle, she thought, that he had even made it to the shop. And come to think of it, his determination to keep his appointment was probably a blessing. Lord knows what would have happened had he gone back inside the house and stayed there.

Now she argued with Berra about what to do next. He wanted to take a shower. She implored him to call Carmen, who was not home, and to get to the hospital. Remembering she had clients waiting for her at the salon, Duke finally decided to leave. On the ride back to the shop, she came up with a number for Larry Berra, the oldest of Yogi's three sons, and told him to contact Carmen immediately and get someone to the house.

Larry reached Carmen on her cell phone, in her car, which at the moment was plugged into a pump at the gas station. "Well," she said, "I can't pull out just yet."

When she finally got home, she, too, was shocked and frightened by the sight of the blood outside and even more so when she saw her husband — a well-groomed sight — sitting in his favorite blue leather chair in the den, holding a compress to his face, watching TV.

"We're going to the hospital," she said.

"I'm going to Old-Timers' Day," he said.

Within a couple of hours, Carmen Berra, no slouch in the face of her husband's legendary stubbornness, finally coaxed him to go to a nearby emergency room. Doctors attended to the cuts and, strangely, sent him home, where blood continued to ooze. The following morning, Carmen convinced him to return, and this time — noticing that Berra was walking stiffly and fearing he had suffered a fracture — the doctors decided to admit him.

Sadly, he was forced to watch Old-Timers' Day on television, fielding get-well calls from a lineup of heavy hitters: Joe Girardi, the manager and former Yankees catcher; Derek Jeter, the beloved captain; Nick Swisher, the congenitally cheerful right fielder. On it went, the lines burning up from the South Bronx, where the collection of former heroes trotted out from the dugout for the first time in eleven years without the greatest of all living Yankees.

Berra wound up stuck in the hospital for almost two excruciating weeks, hating every minute of it. Except for the day Ron Guidry came to visit.

What Guidry initially saw when he knocked on the door and walked inside — Carmen sitting on the edge of the bed, with an expressionless Yogi slumped in a chair, his chin sinking into his chest — was sobering.

"Hey, buddy, how you doing?" Guidry said.

"Gator!" Berra replied, sitting up straighter, calling Guidry by the nickname that always made perfect sense to Yogi, who believed that his friend lived "in the swamps" along with the real gators. His eyes crinkled, and his craggy face broke into an illuminating smile.

Guidry kissed him on the top of his head, and they proceeded to talk for a while about Old-Timers' Day and the coming Hall of Fame weekend, which Guidry was still planning to attend, though less happily now that Berra wasn't going.

"So, Yogi, really, how're you feeling?" Guidry asked.

"All right," he said. "But I can't have no vodka."

More than most, Guidry understood the calamity of the situation. He knew how much Berra relished the few daily ounces — three was the current allowance — that his doctors permitted him to have.

"Not good at all, dude," Guidry said.

Soon a physician arrived to say that the battery of tests they had run on Berra had checked out well. There were just a few minor concerns — residual issues from the fall — that would require him to remain in the hospital for a few more days of therapy and observation.

"Any questions?" the doctor asked.

Guidry decided yes, matter of fact, he did have one.

"And you are?" the doctor asked.

"That's Gator," Berra said, making the informal introduction.

"What about the vodka?" Guidry asked.

"Are you asking if Mr. Berra can have vodka?" she said.

Guidry nodded.

The doctor thought about it for a few seconds and said, "Sure, I don't see why not." When she left the room, Guidry pulled a flask from his pocket. Inside were a few ounces of Ketel One, the Dutch brand Berra insisted on.

"That's for you, buddy," Guidry said.

Berra and Guidry passed the next hour doing what they usually did in each other's company — talking baseball and teasing each other — the storied Yankees pitcher and iconic catcher drawing on an endless reservoir of camaraderie. When it was time for Guidry to go, he leaned close to Berra and said, "See you again in spring training, OK, Yog?"

Berra nodded. Of course he would.

"You'll pick me up at the airport?" he said.

After all these years, did he really have to ask? The answer, Guidry knew, was yes — Berra *had* to ask, over and over, until Guidry was ready to scream.

In the weeks and months ahead, as Berra plotted his Florida journey, his rite of baseball renewal, he would badger Guidry by phone to quiz him on a multitude of arrangements. Carmen, meanwhile, began to have doubts about whether her husband was in any condition to make the trip, to be away from home and from her for weeks on end.

As is often the case with the elderly, the fall had a permanent effect on the man she had been devoted to for six-plus decades, having married him in 1949. The facial cuts had healed, and he was walking again without pain. But he moved more slowly, spoke more softly, and no longer drove or tested the theory that the Jaguar had a protective bubble around it when he was at the wheel.

As spring training drew closer, Carmen picked up the telephone one day, dialed Guidry's number, and found herself on the line with his wife, Bonnie. "Maybe you should tell Ronnie not to be encouraging Yogi to go to Florida," Carmen said, blunt as ever.

Bonnie Guidry didn't quite know how to respond. She and Ron loved the Berras more than anyone they'd known around the Yankees. She considered Carmen a special friend, too. She had gone out in the city with Carmen several times, once taking in a show with Carmen and Yogi's adult granddaughter Lindsay.

Bonnie understood why Carmen was apprehensive. Really, she did. But she also knew how much Yogi loved spring training and how crushing it would be for him not to go, especially this of all years, given the franchise's losses of the previous summer. With Steinbrenner gone, he'd want to be there to help with the healing.

"Carmen," she said, "you know that something could happen to Yogi anywhere. But if anything were to happen in spring training, at least you know he would be doing something he absolutely loves. And you know that Ron will take care of him."

That Carmen did know. That much she could count on.

Waiting by his truck, smoothing his mustache, Guidry wondered what the next few weeks were going to be like. No doubt, he figured, this spring training would be much harder than any previous one.

Berra was going to need more looking after than usual. Ron had spoken to Carmen after the decision had been made that Yogi would come — which, truth be told, Guidry had never doubted.

"You see, his whole world has always revolved around the game, outside of his family," Guidry said. "Baseball has always been his life. It's what the game means to him more than what he means to the game from other people's eyes. But he doesn't look at it that way. He just looks at the damn game, 'cause this is what he knows more about than anything else. And I've always been afraid if you took that away from him, how that would affect him. Because when you take away something from somebody at that age that he loves so much, they may just quit, and I don't want that to happen. Nobody wants that to happen."

Guidry sighed at the mere thought of spring training without Berra — the Yankees without Berra — before pushing it away.

"So I spoke to Carmen about that," he said. "I love her, too, but I wasn't afraid to say, 'You have to let him come.' She didn't get mad, not at all. I think she just knew this is how it's got to be."

Guidry was also a realist; he knew that his friend had aged more in six months than he had over the past six years. The recovery from the fall had required a good deal of inactivity. "When you take a person of his age and you take away six months, it's hard to recuperate and pick up where he left off," he said.

So he waited anxiously for Berra, whose family had prearranged for assistance from the gate to the baggage carousel, where Guidry was supposed to be waiting, or at least had been in the past. He knew that with Berra, if you did something once in a particular way, it had to be done that way for all time.

From outside, peering through the windows, Guidry finally spotted Yogi, a little more slouched than he remembered, looking around for him, already a little flustered. Berra was wearing a blue blazer with an American flag pin on the lapel and a blue-and-white-checked sweater underneath. The coat he would not need in Tampa was draped over his left arm.

Soon Berra was ushered outside by the airline attendant, and his face brightened when he spotted the familiar white truck and Guidry waiting on the sidewalk. Guidry took the bags from the attendant — two moderate-size suitcases, one with the Yankees' familiar interlocking "NY" logo.

"How come you didn't come in?" Berra asked, before proceeding to recite the itinerary for the rest of the day — hotel check-in, shopping, supper, and so on.

Guidry rolled his eyes and complained aloud about what he had gotten himself into by serving as Berra's personal valet.

"Get your ass in the truck," he barked, and Berra giggled like a little boy on his way to his first ballgame. Guidry reached inside for the dark blue baseball cap with the inscription DRIVING MR. YOGI and placed it atop his neatly combed hair. With Guidry at the wheel and Berra in the passenger seat, they pulled into traffic and drove off on another long adventure together, just as they had for eleven glorious years.

2

Roots

Yogi Berra and Ron Guidry first crossed paths in spring training of 1976. Guidry, twenty-five, was trying to build a future for himself as a major-league pitcher before he was too old to be considered a prospect. Berra was a crown jewel of the Yankees' past, returning as Billy Martin's bench coach, the first such appointment in the history of the game. For Berra, it was not love at first sight — or strike.

Sure, Guidry could throw 96 miles per hour, harder than any smallish Yankees pitcher Berra had seen since Lefty Gomez, who retired in 1943. Guidry was two inches short of six feet, weighing in at a touch over 150 pounds — a welterweight after a night of fast-food binging. "But all he had was that fastball," Berra recalled.

Guidry arrived on the scene with so little fanfare that Marty Appel, the team's earnest public relations man, didn't even bother to prepare a mental dossier on him, as he usually did for new players. Appel didn't think Guidry would be around long, and neither did Berra. "Skinny kid . . . maybe a lefty relief specialist . . . nothing real special," Berra remembered thinking.

Guidry had already been up with the Yankees the previous season when Bill Virdon was the manager and the team was in the back end of a two-year stay at Shea Stadium while its own storied ballpark in the South Bronx was being refurbished. When he walked into the clubhouse on May 20, 1975, he immediately got the third degree from two fellow pitchers — Albert Walter Lyle, the bullpen closer otherwise known as "Sparky," and Dick Tidrow, whom teammates called "Dirt."

"What do they call you, 'Ronald'?" Lyle asked.

"Ron, I guess," Guidry said.

"You know," Lyle said, "we don't go around here calling each other by our Christian names."

Guidry gave him an "if you say so" nod.

"So where ya from?" Tidrow asked.

Guidry politely answered that he hailed from Lafayette, Louisiana, where there was considerable water and a lot of snakes and alligators. Though disappointed to hear that the newbie didn't have webbed feet to show them, Tidrow went ahead and christened Guidry with the nickname he would answer to for the rest of his life.

"How's 'Gator'?" he said.

Guidry liked the sound of it and happily went out that day to pitch two scoreless innings in his major-league debut against the Red Sox in the second game of a doubleheader the Sox swept.

After ten appearances in 1975, Guidry was sent to the club's Triple-A Syracuse affiliate when the Yankees broke camp the following spring. He was recalled on May 20, with the Red Sox again in town. When Guidry stepped into Yankee Stadium for the first time, he had "chills and goose bumps that looked like welts" — and he proceeded to absorb a late-game lashing that nearly scarred him forever.

That game is best remembered for a bench-clearing brawl, the result of Yankees teammate Lou Piniella crashing into Carlton Fisk at the plate and then Graig Nettles's body tossing of Boston's flaky left-hander Bill Lee. Nettles separated Lee's shoulder. Guidry was summoned by Martin in the eighth inning with two outs and Boston holding a 4–2 lead.

He got out of the eighth and promptly surrendered four hits and four runs in the ninth, including a two-run homer to Carl Yastrzemski. Ever compassionate and patient with young pitchers, George Steinbrenner bellowed to anyone within half a mile of him that Guidry "didn't have any guts." What Steinbrenner didn't know was that Guidry had pitched out of the Syracuse bullpen four straight days prior to reporting and had asked Martin for a day or two off. Notorious for overusing pitchers, Martin called on him anyway.

Guidry was promptly banished to the bowels of the bullpen and then ordered back to Syracuse several weeks later. Angered by the dismissal, he called Steinbrenner's office, determined to discuss his future. When he received no answer, he got in the car with his wife, Bonnie, and began driving home to Louisiana, convinced that he was wasting his time and would wind up pushing thirty with no career and no means of supporting the child Bonnie was carrying.

About a hundred miles into the trip, somewhere in Pennsylvania on Interstate 80, Bonnie Guidry spoke up: "You've never quit at anything you thought you could do!"

Guidry drove another mile or two, then asked her if she could handle all the uncertainty and packing. Yes, she said. He turned the car around, reported to Syracuse, worked on the hard slider that Lyle had taught him, dominated hitters there, and returned to the Yankees later that summer.

Martin and the coaches could see that he was growing as a pitcher and that he had a quiet determination to succeed. But the shortsighted owner still chafed over Guidry's failure against the Red Sox. That off-season, Steinbrenner lobbied Gabe Paul, his president and general manager, to trade Guidry.

Paul, the independent-thinking architect of what would become Steinbrenner's first pennant and World Series champions, gave him an earful. "I'll agree to it under one condition," he said. "That you issue a press release saying that I, Gabe Paul, unalterably oppose the trade and that you, George Steinbrenner, insist on it, and that when — not if — Ron Guidry becomes an outstanding major-league pitcher for another team, you take the blame."

Startled by Paul's audacity — along with his certainty — Steinbrenner backed off. Even after Guidry had a poor spring training in 1977, Paul wouldn't budge, reminding his boss and others of another late-blooming left-hander named Sandy Koufax.

The 1977 Yankees were defending American League champions, and although they had been swept by Cincinnati's Big Red Machine in the World Series the previous fall, they were an entertaining mix of character and characters. Reggie Jackson was in the room, stirring the drink and a whole lot of controversy. So were Thurman Munson, Catfish Hunter, Lou Piniella, Mickey Rivers — as colorful and cacophonous a cast as there was in baseball at the time. But back inside the clubhouse for the start of the 1977 season, Guidry was much more impressed with a Yankees icon of yore.

Yogi Berra just happened to be in the dressing stall two removed from Guidry's, puffing on a cigarette and pulling up his uniform pants like your average baseball mortal.

Born in 1950, Guidry came of age when Berra was still swinging at pitches over his head or practically on the ground and whacking them with authority. He was the product of an era when a baseball-loving boy, too young to know death from taxes, could at least count on the Yankees playing in the World Series. From the Cajun-rich southwestern region of Louisiana known as Acadiana, Guidry followed them with a growing curiosity alongside his mother, a rabid Yankees fan.

On hot summer Saturday afternoons when the Yankees were on national television, Grace Guidry would summon her son inside for lunch and lock the door so that she could focus on the game without having to worry about where her only child — whom she called "B," short for "Baby" — had run off to.

Before long, Guidry was a fleet young athlete in his own right, running down balls in center field, like Mickey Mantle, the blond matinee idol. He also threw left-handed, pitching in the youth league, and studied Whitey Ford, the great Yankees southpaw, whenever he pitched in a nationally televised game. But to a preadolescent boy not far removed from Saturday morning cartoons, there was something irresistibly folksy—if not flashy—about Yogi Berra, Ford's old catcher, who was so firmly committed to his beloved Yankees that he lugged his aging, squat body out to left field to make way for a younger man behind the plate, Elston Howard.

Guidry was ten when Berra and the Yankees lost game seven of the 1960 World Series to the Pirates in Pittsburgh—considered one of the greatest games ever played. Bill Mazeroski won it for the Pirates when he hit a home run to left field in the ninth inning, a ball that sailed over Berra at his new post and into the stands at Forbes Field. Berra himself hit a three-run homer that day and a hard grounder down the first-base line. First baseman Rocky Nelson fielded the ball and stepped on the bag. Mickey Mantle, who was on first at the time, dove back into the bag ahead of Nelson's tag, barely avoiding a game-ending double play, while the tying run scored.

It never took much prodding for that era's highlights to flood Guidry's mind—the Yankees' defeat of the Reds in the 1961 series and the Giants in 1962, followed by the domination of the Dodgers' Koufax and Don Drysdale in 1963, Berra's last season as a player. In 1964, rookie manager Berra watched helplessly as Cardinals ace Bob Gibson beat his Yankees in game seven.

During his time with the Yankees in 1976, seldom pitching and never sure when the trapdoor to the minors would open and swallow him up, Guidry would walk into the clubhouse and head straight for the row of stalls on the right-hand wall. Lyle had the prime real estate in the corner, Tidrow was next, and then came Guidry, Howard, and Berra.

In his state of major-league limbo, sandwiched between present-day pitchers and yesteryear's catchers, Guidry mostly kept to himself. "I was just a new kid on the block," he said. "You tell everybody hello, but that's about it. You don't walk around strutting your stuff, because you got nothing to strut."

Guidry would occasionally steal a glance to his right in the direction of Howard and Berra, eavesdropping with the hope that he might learn something. He tried to convince himself that he was really a Yankee, just as they were, but that was futile. "I'm looking at Yogi not as a former player but as my *hero*," he said.

Once in a while, Berra would stroll by and ask, "You OK, kid?" To Berra, everyone younger than him was named "kid."

"Yep," Guidry would say, desperately wanting to invite Berra to sit down and share from the vault of pitching wisdom he had collected from the crouch over so many years. Instead, Guidry was deferential to the point of barely rising above mute.

On April 29, with Martin in need of an emergency starter in a home game against the Seattle Mariners, he turned to his quiet southpaw. Guidry responded with 8⅓ innings of shutout ball, 8 strikeouts, and only 2 walks. Lyle closed out the 3–0 victory.

Soon after, Guidry found himself in the rotation, pitching every five days, making a visionary of Gabe Paul, and earning another nickname from Yankees broadcaster Phil Rizzuto. "Louisiana Lightning" became part of the Yankees' nomenclature, and along with it came a totally different clubhouse vibe.

"You start winning games, stopping a losing streak, and your teammates start looking at you in a different light," he said. "You're sitting in the same spot where almost no one said a word to you, but now they're asking you little stuff."

How's your arm?

Hey, Gator, want a sandwich?

Need a coffee?

Guidry looked at the others differently as well, especially Berra. He began to feel more involved and entitled.

"Now that I'm earning my stripes and I'm starting to think maybe I can say something to him," Guidry said. "I'm telling myself, 'You know what, he's not playing anymore, and if he wants to get another World Series opportunity, he may actually be thinking that I'm a guy who might help him.' I'm thinking that maybe this is how it all works, so if I say something to him, he'll want to talk to me."

But not necessarily on cue.

"You got Munson over there, one of the best catchers in baseball," Berra replied to one of Guidry's early entreaties.

Guidry persisted, convinced that Berra was only trying to push him closer to Munson, the all-star, and not brushing him off.

"What you start to realize is that he's not that open a person, especially with ordinary people," Guidry said. "But we're not ordinary people; we're teammates. And he's sitting there, and he's starting to see in my face that I really want to ask these things, because I know there's never been any question that's ever been asked that he doesn't know something about. He's seen it all, done it all, so he starts to think, *Here we go again, just like with Whitey Ford and Mel Stottlemyre, another young guy who maybe I can help.*"

So Guidry, before facing the imposing lineup of the Kansas City Royals in mid-June, looked over at Berra and blurted out, "Jesus Christ, George Brett is smokin'—how the hell are we getting him out?"

Puffing away on a cigarette, Berra looked up, impressed by Guidry's choice of pronoun.

"Go up and in, first pitch, see what he does, send a message," he said. "Then you got opportunities."

"Shit," Guidry said, "you want me to go up and in on George Brett on the first pitch?"

"Yeah, that's right," Berra said. "And then he'll look at you, like, *You're coming up and in on* me? You give him a look right back: *Don't take it personal, pal. I'm just figuring out a way to get you out.*"

Berra smiled, impishly. "Then you give him a slider away."

The next day, Guidry pitched a three-hit shutout against the Royals. As he had been told, Guidry went inside right away on Brett, who went hitless. "I'm thinking, hmmm, we got something here," he said.

He was fascinated by how matter-of-factly the advice rolled off Berra's tongue, as if he'd dropped a quarter into a slot for a candy bar. Berra was not an eloquent man, and not very talkative either. But when he did have his say, he was direct, each word having a purpose.

The more they spoke, the more Guidry realized that Yogi Berra's reputation as a man who made language a misadventure was just window-dressing. "You can't be like Yogi and have no smarts," Guidry said. "Life doesn't work like that. What I was finding out there was that Yogi was really smart when it came to something he cared about. Now, did he care about gardening, about food critics? No, he didn't. So when, with everyday people, he doesn't have anything to talk about, maybe people think he's not intelligent. But when it's a bunch of baseball players and it's about the game, he could talk to them all night. And there's nobody smarter."

There was, he learned, a glorious simplicity to Berra's logic, and also a limit. Guidry could ask a thousand questions, and Berra's answers would all be variations on his time-honored philosophy: *Don't think too much*. In so many words, he would advise Guidry just to figure out what a guy couldn't hit—fastball rising in the zone, slider in on the hands or breaking down and away—and throw it. You get a hitter who can't hit a breaking ball, why the hell are you going to throw him a fastball? Make him *learn* to hit that pitch, and when he does, try the other one.

"It's a game of back and forth, back and forth," Berra would tell him, over and over. To twenty-first-century sabermetricians, this might sound like pop psychology for Little Leaguers. But consider the context: in a place where a young pitcher felt the gaze of Steinbrenner upon him whenever he wound up, and therefore the weight of his career upon his back, Berra's uncomplicated approach was profoundly reassuring. It made even more sense when Guidry began mowing down major-league hitters with surprising regularity.

"I threw two pitches, fastball and slider, so it was fifty-fifty," he said. "Well, Yogi's thing was to knock off fifty percent of the guessing game, not for the hitter but for me." On the way to winning sixteen games against seven defeats in 1977, Guidry became the X factor in a one-hundred-win season that was barely good enough to hold off the Red Sox and Orioles in the American League East.

But there was more to learn from the neighboring legend during that stormy season when the Bronx was literally burning, when Mount St. Steinbrenner was continually erupting, when Billy Martin and Reggie Jackson were frequently squabbling. Ron Guidry was evolving into a full-fledged Yankee. How to act like one while surviving inside the team's increasingly chaotic universe was the next item on the agenda.

Things came to a head on June 18, 1977, in a game against the Red Sox at Fenway Park. Although Guidry had been a Yankee for less than two years, he had already come to expect the unexpected at the sight of the Yankees' divisional rivals.

On this Saturday afternoon, in front of a national television audience, the Yankees were getting their heads handed to them by the potent Red Sox lineup. In the sixth inning of an ultimate 10–4 defeat, Boston's Jim Rice looped a ball into short right field. Reggie Jackson, playing deep for the right-handed slugger with good power to the opposite field, came in to field the ball after it had landed in the grass. He had misjudged its depth — or so he would later claim.

In Martin's steadfast opinion, Rice had wound up on second base only because Jackson had loafed on the play. To Martin, an average talent who had succeeded as a player because he wouldn't take no for an answer, not hustling was an unpardonable major-league sin. No fan of Jackson's to begin with, Martin decided he had seen enough of his pitcher *and* his right fielder. Before he went out to the mound to remove his starter, Mike Torrez, he told reserve outfielder Paul Blair to pick up his glove and get out to right field.

Jackson was incredulous when he saw Blair coming his way. He had never been removed from the field during a game before, and he believed that Martin, frustrated by how the game was going, was taking it out on him. Much worse, Jackson also believed that Martin's general treatment of him was in no small part racially based — an opinion he articulated to reporters soon after.

In the dugout, Guidry, sitting next to Martin's trusted pitching coach, Art Fowler, watched the potential train wreck unfold. With his stock rising fast, Guidry had become something of the class pet, required by Fowler to sit by his side between starts. That gave him a front-row seat for the spectacle about to take place.

Here came Jackson jogging in, smoke billowing from his ears, heading straight for Martin, who had already returned to the dugout and positioned himself in the corner right where Jackson would be descending the steps. But before Jackson arrived, the Yankees' coaching police, in the persons of Berra and Howard, were moving into lockdown position — "like a movie scene, where the actors get up according to the script without saying a word," Guidry said.

With Martin champing at the bit to take on Jackson, Berra and Howard had to move tactically and in tandem — two great catchers, Guidry noted, trained to foresee the possibilities of the game from the best seat in the ballpark.

"That's what was so amazing," Guidry said, "those two guys actually knew something was going to happen soon as Billy said, 'Blair, get your glove.' They both stood up. They had the smarts to know that this doesn't look good, something's going to happen here, I need to be ready. Nobody else did, just them. Me, I'm just sitting there on my butt, never even thought about getting up."

Actually, the thought did cross Guidry's mind as Jackson ran in from right field that maybe it was time for a physical altercation between Jackson and Martin. The two had been verbally sparring from the beginning of 1977, Jackson's first season in New York. Maybe punches were inevitable — and preferable for everyone involved.

"At that moment, if you asked me, I would've said that we should have just let the sons of bitches go," he said. "Here are two guys that don't get along with each other, that's obvious. And now this has happened and Reggie's like, *You challenged my honor, you slapped me in the face, let's take it out back and handle it.*"

The truth was that Howard was not much more enamored of Jackson than Martin was. Howard was the first African American to play for the Yankees, debuting in 1955, or eight long years after Jackie Robinson broke the color line. However belatedly, Howard had integrated baseball's most powerful franchise with a proud and quiet dignity. Given that, he didn't understand or appreciate Jackson's habit of calling attention to himself.

Nor did Berra, who loved to tell the story of how his good friend "Ellie" had once deflated Jackson after Reggie had asked Berra and Howard how he would have fit in on the great Yankees teams of the fifties and sixties. "Fifth outfielder," deadpanned Howard, which Berra thought was comically brilliant.

If Berra had no patience for Jackson's shtick, he did have an abiding respect for his big stick. As a longtime clubhouse kibitzer, he also enjoyed how Jackson unintentionally made himself the butt of his associates' teasing, even long after he retired. For example, when he was asked to throw out the ceremonial first pitch of the 2008 season at Yankee Stadium, Jackson asked Berra to accompany him to the mound. Berra didn't really want to but reluctantly agreed.

In the dugout, he muttered, "Why the hell does he want me out there with him?"

Standing nearby, Derek Jeter cracked, "Yog, it's because he doesn't want to get booed."

Whatever their personal feelings that day in the visitors' dugout at Fenway Park, Berra and Howard had their priorities straight — first and foremost, they were Yankees. And they had a game to play and a pennant to win. They intuitively knew that Martin or Jackson — or both — could do serious damage to the other, not to mention the ball club. Martin was much older and smaller but was a notorious brawler who was known for landing punches on his own players and living to brag about it. Outweighed by sixty pounds, he wasn't backing off as Jackson hopped down the steps and got right in his chest.

"You never wanted me on this team in the first place," Jackson said.

"I ought to kick your ass," Martin replied.

"Billy was real furious," Berra said. "There was no telling what he was going to do."

Meanwhile, Ray Negron — a young clubhouse assistant and a protégé of Steinbrenner's — tried to cut off the television audience by putting a towel over the camera closest to the dugout. But nothing of physical consequence really happened, mainly because Berra and Howard were on the job, reacting on muscle memory in the way they had once backed up first base to keep an errant throw by an infielder from rolling into the dugout.

As strong as Jackson was, there was no chance he was going to escape Howard's grip, Guidry said. Not that time or later that season when the Yankees were celebrating winning the American League pennant and Jackson got a little too carried away, spraying a bottle of champagne into Howard's eyes. Howard picked him up like a large potted plant and evicted him from his space.

As for Berra, he was much stronger than anyone imagined, Guidry said. Martin struggled to break free from Berra's grip, nearly falling onto the bench, but to no avail. "Once that little guy gets his monkey claws on you, you ain't goin' nowhere," Guidry said, vouching for Berra's ability, even well into his seventies, to hold a person in place with a firm grip of the shoulder or wrist.

"My point is, you learned that this guy was physical," Guidry said. "You realized that Billy, tough a guy as he was, wasn't getting away from Yogi, same as Reggie with Ellie. And by doing what they did, in a moment when the rest of us just sat there and watched, you realize now how smart they were and what might have happened had they not been."

Across the years, Berra and Guidry would share a laugh whenever the near brawl came up — not that Berra was inclined to expound on his role in stopping it. That wasn't his style, and at least with Guidry, what was the point?

"We all were there; we all saw it," Guidry said. "But the big thing is that Yogi and Ellie, they knew it wasn't just us. You had millions of people sitting at home watching it around the country. And when you look back, you have to ask yourself, 'Is that how you really would have wanted the world to see how we are?'"

To the young Ron Guidry, it was a career lesson that he would never forget: how a Yankee acts and comes through in the clutch.

Despite all the chaos that year, the Yankees went on to beat Brett and the Royals in the 1977 American League Championship Series (ALCS). Then they trounced the Dodgers in the World Series, which climaxed with three Jackson home runs in game six.

But 1978 would prove to be Guidry's year to shine. He was virtually unhittable, Koufax reincarnated. With total command of his slider, he won his first 13 decisions, compiled a 25–3 record with a 1.74 earned run average (ERA), and had 9 shutouts and an 18-strikeout game against the Angels on June 17.

He was the unanimous winner of the American League Cy Young Award and runner-up to Jim Rice for MVP. It was one of the greatest pitching seasons in baseball history, and yet early in the season, Guidry still wanted to pick Berra's brain.

He didn't approach Berra every day, just now and then, until one day Berra gave Guidry a look that told him enough was enough. The exact time and nature of the question are lost in the blur of years, but it was somewhere along the way to Guidry's first thirteen wins.

How many times did he have to be told what he already knew? Wasn't it always the same advice?

Look, kid, you did it. You figured it out. I can't help you no more.

"Well, there comes a time where you know that you got to stop asking questions," Guidry said. "I mean, he wasn't upset, he wasn't mad, he was just being Yogi. But the way that he answered it, I got the impression that he was saying, *You're ten and oh, twelve and oh, whatever, what the hell more do you want?* At least that's what I got from it, just the way I felt."

Mostly, Guidry felt obliged to Berra, and would for the rest of his days. He would always credit Sparky Lyle for the slider and Dick Tidrow for helping him with pure pitching mechanics. But no one, he said, ever made the mental part of the game as easy as Berra.

Don't think too much. "Probably the best advice anyone ever gave me," he said.

The Yankees won another World Series, beating the Dodgers again in 1978, but as the years passed, the team would more and more be defined by organizational chaos and change. Managers would come and go, come back and go again. With few exceptions, the pitching staff revolved like the front door at Macy's. Thurman Munson's death in the pilot's seat of his private plane in August 1979 cast a years-long pall over the franchise.

For Guidry, bridging the decades and generations, there was always comfort in the reliability of Berra nearby—sitting in his underwear, puffing on a cigarette or chewing tobacco—when the latest Yankee-land news broke. Berra was always a clubhouse newshound, and when he returned as a coach in 1976, he took to calling Marty Appel daily for about ten minutes' worth of inside dope. With Steinbrenner running things, there was never a shortage.

Although Berra was no longer his philosophical guru, Guidry still considered him more mentor than friend. "You know, I can't get too close to him as a coach," he said. "You can talk, but you can't develop a real close relationship, because he might have to drop a hammer on you one day. But as a coach on our club, he wasn't a man you had to walk by and bow to all the time."

If not one of the guys, Berra—with a finger on the pulse of a team that was always on edge about one thing or another—served as a shrewd liaison for the manager. On plane rides, he would work his way to the back, where the core veterans—Guidry, Piniella, Goose Gossage—were holding court. He'd share a round and let them be.

In 1984, Berra's life as a Yankee turned dramatically when Steinbrenner made him manager, reveling in the appointment of a legend and then proceeding to torture him as he did all the others.

In early April, after opening the season in Kansas City, Berra began to realize what he had gotten himself into. Guidry would never forget Berra's ashen face when the Boss ordered the young shortstop Bobby Meacham to the minors after he'd committed a two-out error in a 7–6 loss to the Rangers in the fourth game of the season. The often incomprehensible pressures of the job only mounted from there.

What stuck in Guidry's craw was how Berra was constantly measured by Steinbrenner, the media, and fans against Martin, as if Berra and Martin were working with the same quality of players. By that standard, Berra was in a no-win situation from day one.

So much of the irascible core talent of the championship teams — Rivers, Jackson, Nettles, Chris Chambliss, Munson, and Hunter — was long gone. Worse for Guidry was the misery of a sore-armed season — 10–11 with a 4.51 ERA — that kept him from possibly making a difference for the man who had helped him so much.

"Now we're trying to patchwork it, signing old players who have names but can't do the job anymore," Guidry said. "And then we had just gone through that era of winning all the time, and so there are expectations that you have to do that every year.

"But if Yogi had had what Billy had, he would have done the same job. We played hard for Billy, but we all knew that his hardest job besides dealing with the Reggie thing and George was filling out the lineup."

It was painful for Guidry to watch Berra in the crosshairs during an 87–75 third-place season — smoking more than he should have been and once so infuriated by Steinbrenner's second-guessing that he threw a pack of cigarettes at the Boss. *You make out the damn lineup if you're so smart.*

"George actually tried once, but he couldn't do anything with it," Guidry said. "It got to the point where you wanted to do something to help Yogi, but you couldn't. You felt helpless."

There were lighter moments, the kind Berra was so good at generating, intentionally or otherwise. On the same night that Meacham was sent to the minors, Guidry's family visited from Lafayette, as they often did when the Yankees played in Arlington. His father, Roland, would mark the occasion by preparing a rabbit-stew feast, Cajun-style. Like a student placing an apple on his teacher's desk, Guidry would bring some into the clubhouse for his favorite coaches, Berra and Howard, no strings attached. But this time, Roland Guidry made a special request: he wanted to know if there was any chance that Ron's teenage brother could meet Yogi Berra.

Travis Guidry had been born eighteen years after Ron. Deprived of oxygen during a difficult birth, he was brain-damaged. Ron made no promises but said he would ask.

During batting practice, Roland noticed his son chatting with Berra near second base and gesturing to the area behind third base. As Berra began walking toward them with Ron alongside him, Roland grabbed Travis to move down the aisle. But a few feet from the barrier in front, the path was blocked by a gaggle of fans with visions of an autograph.

When Ron saw his father's head poking through the crowd, he yelled, "Where's Travis?" Roland pointed and shrugged. At this point, Berra reached out his arms and yelled, "Let that boy through." A pathway formed, and within seconds Berra's arm was around Travis Guidry, who went home with a hug and a handshake he never forgot. Berra was compensated with the gratitude of the Guidry family, the depth of which he would not understand until years later.

Steinbrenner's antics aside, there were plenty of laughs in the dugout that season. During one game, the Yankees were down a run in the middle innings with a man on first and nobody out. Would Berra bunt the runner into scoring position? The man who had spent his career with a team famous for clutch, power hitting had never been enamored of small ball. Berra flashed the hit sign.

The next inning, same situation, and now the players were anticipating the sacrifice again. No dice. From his seat on the bench, Guidry glanced down the line and could see some of his teammates looking around in bewilderment.

Suddenly a voice — Guidry couldn't remember whose: "Skip, don't you think you should make a move?"

Without turning his head, Berra took one side step to the left. "How's that?" he said, setting off a round of convulsive laughter.

But it wasn't funny when the end came for Berra, an absurd sixteen games into the 1985 season. Steinbrenner had promised at the outset of spring training to let Berra be, not make a change for the whole season. Instead, he fired him on April 28 after the White Sox finished off a three-game sweep in Chicago that left the Yankees with a 6–10 record.

Steinbrenner cited "a lack of discipline," while adding that he'd agonized over the firing and hadn't slept the night before announcing it. The worst part was that Steinbrenner — who had, as always, made the decision unilaterally — didn't even deliver the news himself, leaving it to his general manager, Clyde King, to tell Berra that Billy Martin would be returning for a fourth turn, as Steinbrenner's eleventh manager in his twelve years as owner. Although Steinbrenner did call Berra the next day at home, it was a terrible demonstration by the Boss, one that Berra would not soon forgive or forget.

When the news spread in the clubhouse, the emerging star, Don Mattingly, was particularly irate. Their anger simmering, the veterans Willie Randolph, Dave Winfield, and Don Baylor refused to comment, although Baylor's attempt to kick a clubhouse trash can all the way to Indiana said it all.

Berra remained in the manager's office with the door closed for half an hour after the game. His son Dale, who had been acquired in a trade with Pittsburgh during the off-season, was with him. When they emerged, Dale's face was tearstained. His father told him not to worry; he'd be on the golf course back home in New Jersey by Monday afternoon. "Play hard for Billy, and you'll be fine," he said.

Then he told reporters, referring to Steinbrenner, "He's the boss. He can do what he wants."

As the players left Comiskey Park and filed onto the bus for the ride from Chicago's South Side to O'Hare International Airport, they were stunned to find Berra in his customary seat in the front. What the hell? he figured. He was going to the airport, too. Why take a cab when he already had a ride?

"It was hard to believe that he was taking the bus with us," Dale Berra said. "But that was Dad, showing his humanity, wanting everything to feel as normal as possible."

How many men, he wondered, could have instantly processed those warring emotions and compartmentalized their fury, saving it for the man upstairs? He remembered his older brother Tim once telling him how Howard Schnellenberger had responded when he was fired three games into Tim's one-year fling with the Baltimore Colts. *He stormed off swearing and raging, right past the players, without so much as a goodbye.*

During the quiet, somber ride, Berra stayed in his seat, saying nothing until the bus rolled to its first terminal stop, his place to get off. He stood up and turned around to the players. In a few words, he thanked them, wished them luck, and told them to keep working hard. An awkward moment of silence was followed by a heartfelt round of applause.

With a wave, Berra stepped down to the curb and retrieved his bag from underneath the bus. The driver climbed back aboard, the door closed, and the bus pulled away. Dale was in tears as he glimpsed his father's familiar hunched figure through the window.

Guidry watched all of this unfold in his own emotional vortex, the veteran in him knowing this was the flip side of glory, the cold-hearted exit most people in the game—himself included—were likely to make. Still, it was Yogi Berra being discarded from the bus like excess baggage, an old piece of furniture left by the curb. For a moment, he wanted to cry, but he didn't. The guys were all around. The bus rolled on. There was a plane to catch to the next town.

The emotion passed. But Guidry would not forget it.

3

The Late Show

In the late afternoon shadows of winter, the day cold but precipitation-free, a black town car was about to whisk George Steinbrenner from Newark Airport and take him on what may have been the longest ride of his sixty-eight years — and certainly the longest in the fourteen years since he had fired Yogi Berra.

At the curb, Steinbrenner handed a small garment bag to the driver and slipped into the back seat next to Rick Cerrone, the Yankees' director of media operations, in his fourth year of serving Steinbrenner's promotional and emotional whims 24-7. Something seemed different about the Boss today. He lacked his customary bombast, wearing a sad-sack frown on a face that normally radiated vitality. As the driver worked the maze of airport roadways, Steinbrenner barely said a word, which Cerrone knew didn't happen often.

Also odd was his choice of dress: Steinbrenner had eschewed what Cerrone liked to call his "power blue" for a decidedly neutral camel-colored sports coat and beige turtleneck. Cerrone recalled reading somewhere that the last thing a leveraged businessman should ever do is show up to an important meeting wearing off colors bordering on brown.

Leverage was the underlying issue of this rare occasion. Steinbrenner, a man steeped in power and privilege, had no leverage. Could the bland look have been an unwitting admission of his predicament — heading for a meeting he had already ceded control of?

Cerrone considered the call he had received in his Yankee Stadium office from the Tampa-based Boss only a few weeks earlier, when the possibility of the journey north for a years-overdue meeting with Yogi Berra, a Yankees immortal, was broached. "What do you think about me doing this?" Steinbrenner had said.

"I think it's terrific," Cerrone had replied.

Somehow, this advice had only agitated Steinbrenner, as if he'd hoped to be talked out of it. "Of course you're going to say that," he'd barked. "You're his friend."

Well, that's a stretch, Cerrone had thought, although admittedly he had been around Berra a fair number of times, was a great fan, and once, while working for the baseball commissioner's office, had asked Berra to autograph the famous 1984 *Sports Illustrated* cover of old number 8 from behind, with the headline YOGI'S BACK (as in back to managing the Yankees).

"What should I write?" Berra had asked.

"How about 'It ain't over 'til it's over'?" Cerrone had said.

Berra had nodded and written, "Best Wishes."

Of course, he wasn't back for long — one season plus sixteen games. Fourteen years later, the tables were turned, and Steinbrenner was, for perhaps the first time in his life, unsure about what he wanted to do, or what he should do.

"George, I'm giving you my best counsel," Cerrone had said on the phone. "I think it would be a great thing for you to do, and it would be great for the Yankees."

Finally, Steinbrenner had said, "OK, I'll do it. But you're going with me."

Unsure how he should feel about that, Cerrone eventually settled on the position that Steinbrenner had demonstrated great trust in his professional judgment. Cerrone was no ballplayer — like Rick Cerone, the former Yankees catcher with the same name minus one *r* — but he, too, was a team player.

The appointment was set for 5:00 P.M., and Steinbrenner, in deference to the famously punctual man waiting on him, did not want to be late. As he sometimes did in advance of important events, he had ordered his driver to make trial runs to their destination from the airport to determine the fastest route. Naturally, it was impossible to simulate early-rush-hour congestion, especially in densely populated north Jersey. They soon found themselves in slowing traffic on the Garden State Parkway.

Steinbrenner repeatedly checked his watch, while looking out the window and tapping his foot. Cerrone had never seen him so nervous. "The word that comes to mind is 'trepidation,'" he said.

Traffic eased, and the town car made its way off the parkway and into a back-area parking lot on the hilly campus of Montclair State University. It rolled to a stop in front of a new minor-league ballpark next to a small, gleaming building. Steinbrenner pushed open the car door, got out and stood up straight, and was led to the building's rear entrance.

There he stood face-to-face with the smaller, bespectacled man who had assiduously avoided him for almost fourteen years. It was about ten minutes after five when Steinbrenner arrived at Berra's doorstep, in effect to thank the self-exiled Yankees great for having made this day necessary.

Berra looked at his humbled ex-boss and tapped his watch. "You're late," he grumped.

The mood momentarily lightened, or so Steinbrenner thought, so he feigned exasperation. "Yogi, gimme a break. I came all the way from Florida!"

Other than a passing nod at the funerals of Billy Martin in 1989 and Mickey Mantle in 1995, this was the first direct communication between the two men since 1985.

• • •

How George Steinbrenner came face-to-face with Yogi Berra in a back-campus corner on January 5, 1999, is a tale of journalistic and entertainment enterprise buttressed by a fair amount of determined arm-twisting.

The campus sports complex was the public-private brainstorm of a handful of Montclair-area power brokers who had united under the organizational heading Friends of Yogi Inc. With $10 million in funding provided by the private company of Floyd Hall, a Montclair resident and Kmart's chief executive, and the New Jersey Educational Facilities Authority, a 3,900-seat ballpark called Yogi Berra Stadium was built to house an independent minor-league franchise along with the university's team.

Someone in the group had another idea that was fine by Berra, who had come to a time in his life when a legacy beyond long-yellowed press clippings had begun to matter. To the quaint little ballpark, his incorporated friends added a modest museum to display his trove of memorabilia and serve as a north Jersey baseball hub and developmental center for youth-oriented educational programs.

The groundbreaking for the complex occurred in April 1997, and the opening of the Yogi Berra Museum & Learning Center was set for December 1998. Hoping for a timely promotional blast, Dave Kaplan, the museum's newly hired director and former *New York Daily News* Sunday sports editor, contacted WFAN, the city's all-sports talk powerhouse, and offered the museum (and Berra by extension) for a live broadcast.

Suzyn Waldman was the station's Yankees reporter, who during the off-season hosted an evening show on weeknights following the popular afternoon drive-time tandem of Mike (Francesa) and the Mad Dog (Chris Russo). Waldman was thrilled to take her show on the road and quickly came up with a timely theme. As 1998 marked the twenty-fifth anniversary of the Mets winning the 1973 National League pennant, she would do a tribute show with the manager of that team, Yogi Berra.

"I was going to do the show from six to nine, with Yogi and some of the ex-Mets in the studio or on the phone," Waldman said.

Mark Chernoff, the station's executive producer, thought of a deliciously audacious alternative. He asked Waldman, "Wouldn't it be cool if you could get Yogi and George to reunite on the show?"

Yes, it would be amazing, she replied. But so would picking up the phone and asking Steinbrenner if she could pitch on Opening Day for the Yankees.

To begin with, several people — Gene Michael, who had served Steinbrenner in several organizational roles, and Arthur Richman, an old PR hand, to name just two — had already implored Steinbrenner to do whatever he could to return Berra to Yankee Stadium. But even if Steinbrenner could be convinced to participate in an arranged and very public peacemaking, everyone knew that Berra was resolute about not having anything to do with the Yankees for as long as Steinbrenner owned them.

After the 1985 firing, he had, as promised, filled his days by playing golf, working out, and spending time with his grandchildren. But at age sixty, while he wasn't much interested in the eventual sad state the Yankees fell into, he was far from finished with baseball. The game was his life; it was in his blood. By 1986, he was back coaching, this time with the Houston Astros, at the behest of his Montclair neighbor and team owner John McMullen. It was McMullen who had famously said of his minority ownership role with Steinbrenner's Yankees, "There's nothing more limited than being a limited partner of George Steinbrenner."

Over time, there were numerous opportunities for Berra to return to Yankee Stadium, including a 1988 ceremony in which he and his mentor, Bill Dickey, were officially given plaques in Monument Park. No, thank you, Yogi had said. He also had declined an invitation to his best friend Phil Rizzuto's fiftieth wedding anniversary celebration at the stadium in 1993.

Many members of the media and fans on the street applauded his stand. *Daily News* columnist Mike Lupica called him the one man

Steinbrenner could not buy. Don Mattingly, who had grown into superstardom under Berra, said, "All I can say is, it is a deep profound joy that Yogi won't sell out. The man has character. He has pride."

But others would occasionally advise him in print and in passing to abandon his grudge, if only to send the message that the Yankees were ultimately about the men in uniform and not the man upstairs. Whitey Ford told him to forget about George, just come back, the people want to see you — heck, *we* want to see you.

Even Carmen Berra would tell her husband from time to time that enough was enough. "No," he would say, "I'm keeping my word. I don't care what anyone says. I'm not going back as long as he's there."

No one could persuade him otherwise. During the 1996 season, Joe Torre's first in New York, he would call from time to time to solicit Berra's thoughts on his coalescing band of Yankees. Berra told him that he loved the young Derek Jeter's professionalism and the fiery Paul O'Neill's perfectionism. He was already touting the hard-throwing Mariano Rivera, then setting up for John Wetteland, as a future star.

"Then come in the clubhouse and meet the guys," Torre said.

"I'm rooting for you; I'm always a Yankee," Berra said. "But I'll watch from home."

Torre tried again after the Yankees won the 1996 World Series, appealing to Berra's partiality for championship festivities, given his thirteen-ring collection (ten as a player and three as a coach). "Yog, I'd be honored if you would present me my ring," he said.

"Joe, I can't," Berra said, and left it at that.

Steinbrenner had good reason to believe the rift was beyond repair, having invited Berra to attend many Old-Timers' Days, among other stadium events, but always through intermediaries. That was the stumbling block that Steinbrenner could never avoid. He didn't comprehend that Berra's self-banishment had never been about being fired, only the Boss's callous execution.

As a dedicated lifer, Berra accepted baseball's axiomatic realities, understanding that managers were hired to be fired. If he hadn't, he never would have returned to the Yankees after being fired in 1964, long before anyone had heard of Steinbrenner. All Berra had done as a rookie manager that year (he'd retired as a player the previous season) was win ninety-nine games and take the team to the seventh game of the World Series.

But Berra had a tough decision to make before that seventh game. Whitey Ford was suffering from a circulation problem in his left shoulder, so Berra had to choose someone of inferior ability or pitch the rookie Mel Stottlemyre on two days' rest against Bob Gibson. Stottlemyre had come up from the minors in August to go 9–3 with a 2.06 earned run average. He had won game one of the series against Gibson. Berra believed in the rookie and his sinkerball, so he walked up to Stottlemyre the day before the game and said, "Kid, you got the ball."

It didn't work out, as Stottlemyre left with shoulder stiffness in the fifth inning, trailing 3–0. The Cardinals took the series, and general manager Ralph Houk blamed Berra—forgetting that he had gone into the series without the services of his best reliever, Pedro Ramos—and fired him with the excuse that he hadn't been able to control a ninety-nine-win team. In a bizarre turn of events, Houk hired Johnny Keane, the manager who had just beaten them, and the 1965 Yankees plunged to sixth place on the way to bottoming out completely. Even then, Berra demonstrated a knack for moving on, crossing over into Queens and becoming a Met. It wasn't long before he was back in the World Series, coaching for Gil Hodges in 1969. That was the season the miracle Mets shocked the Baltimore Orioles and all of baseball. When Hodges died unexpectedly in 1972, Berra was again named manager. That summer, the Yankees retired his number 8 on Old-Timers' Day. But Berra was busy. He sent his son Larry in his place.

The Mets fired him, too, less than two years after his team lost the 1973 World Series to Reggie Jackson and the Oakland A's. At the time, he had a winning record, but only marginally.

When Carmen would remind Yogi over the years that Steinbrenner hadn't been the only owner who "didn't treat you properly," he would shrug and say, "That was part of the game."

Berra was remarkably consistent about his feelings from 1985 to 2011. "Getting fired didn't really bother me," he said, looking back. "You work for George, you know the deal. He changes managers all the time. What bothered me was the lack of respect. To me that was unforgivable."

In his mind, the decision of who deserved to be in the dugout was always ownership's prerogative, record notwithstanding. But there was an appropriate way to make such changes and an inappropriate way, and one was easily distinguishable from the other.

For example, when the Mets fired him, owner M. Donald Grant called the house and got Carmen on the phone. "It looks like we're going to have to let Yogi go," he told her.

"You have to give him a little more time," she said, not necessarily pleading for another chance, merely the opportunity for her husband to make a more graceful exit. Her mother was visiting from St. Louis, and an immediate dismissal would have been embarrassing for him.

Grant said he understood. He waited two weeks and called back to ask if it was a better time. "He was a gentleman about it," Carmen said. "So in Yogi's mind, that was OK."

Given the stubborn nature of the principals and the trenches Berra and Steinbrenner were dug into, Waldman wasn't brimming with optimism when she called the Boss. In her years covering the Yankees as a radio reporter—before she would become part of their radio broadcast team with John Sterling—she had developed a close professional relationship with the Boss. An admitted chauvinist, Steinbrenner respected Waldman's baseball knowledge and her passion for the game. He trusted her to the point that he granted her a live and uproarious interview on her show upon his return to baseball in 1993 following a two-year ban by Commissioner Fay Vincent for a sinister scheme to sully the reputation of his star outfielder, Dave Winfield.

"I want to talk to you about Yogi," Waldman said when Steinbrenner picked up.

"What's wrong?" he said with alarm.

"Nothing," she said. "I just think it's time you two got back to-gether."

He was quiet for a few moments.

"OK," he said. "Maybe we'll try to do something during spring training."

She told him that wasn't what she had in mind, and on top of that, it would snow in Tampa before Berra would show up at the Yankees' complex.

At that point, Waldman was appealing to Steinbrenner without even knowing if Berra would agree. Like most people whose time around the Yankees began while Berra was in exile, she had no rela-tionship with him, had never met him until Phil and Cora Rizzuto had introduced her to him at the funeral of Mel Allen, the former "Voice of the Yankees," in 1996.

But her conversation with Steinbrenner left her hopeful. While Steinbrenner groused about a December voyage to New Jer-sey — "What if it snows or there's an ice storm?" he asked — there was one thing she knew from experience: if he wasn't at all open to it, he would have said no and hung up. When he argued, that was a good sign.

Maybe, she started to believe, the timing was right. After an eigh-teen-year absence from the top, the Yankees were well into a dynastic run — four World Series titles in five years beginning with the arrival of Torre and Derek Jeter in 1996. And Steinbrenner was pushing sev-enty, becoming more of a softie with each passing year. He had even considered selling the team to the Dolan family, owners of Cablevi-sion and Madison Square Garden.

The previous summer, he had buried the hatchet with another long-absent (though far less prominent) member of the Yankees family. After reading an emotional appeal by Jim Bouton's son in the *New York Times*, Steinbrenner had invited the banished former pitcher — whose best-selling *Ball Four* had spilled baseball's behav-ioral secrets and made him something of a pariah — for Old-Timers'

Day. The Boss also had sobbed on national television after the Yankees swept the San Diego Padres in the 1998 World Series, wrapping up a record 125-win season (playoffs included).

Steinbrenner called it the perfect season except for one thing: "There was a missing piece," he said, and that piece was Berra.

While his storied franchise was bigger and financially more successful than ever, it was a difficult time for the extended Yankees family. Mel Allen's death in June 1996 followed the excruciating passing of Mickey Mantle the year before. By the time Waldman called Steinbrenner about Berra, he knew that Joe DiMaggio was down to his final swings in his battle with lung cancer.

After DiMaggio's death in March 1999, or about three months after Steinbrenner's journey to Jersey, a well-known podiatrist and close DiMaggio friend named Rock Positano told the *New York Daily News* that DiMaggio had been responsible for Steinbrenner's willingness to go to Berra, hat in hand. According to Positano, during a forty-five-minute visit at Memorial Regional Hospital in Hollywood, Florida, DiMaggio had told Steinbrenner, "It shouldn't be a personal thing. It should be first for the fans, then for the game, then for the Yankees."

This all sounded like another stirring chapter in Yankees history — a dying DiMaggio lecturing the inscrutable Steinbrenner. Except there was no reason to believe — and there was no acknowledgment from Steinbrenner — that DiMaggio's lecture ever happened. More likely it was another attempt to mythologize Joe D., never known to be an advocate for the fans or, for that matter, the franchise.

Most people chose to believe that Steinbrenner's gesture proved once and for all that he had a big heart buried beneath the bluster; that he intuitively knew it was time to act on Berra and merely needed the right set of circumstances. Others wondered if it was more calculated, the Boss's kinder, gentler side finding common ground with his business interests. If ever there was a time the Yankees brand needed a grand gesture, this was it.

"Maybe it was because people were dying around him and he was getting older himself," Waldman said. "I can't really speak to that. But whatever people may or may not think, the Yogi thing bothered him, at least for as long as I had known him. That was one thing in his life that he was not happy about."

Still, even after agreeing to make the trip, there remained the vexing issue of how this was all going to unfold and what role Steinbrenner was supposed to play. "What exactly does he want me to do?" the Boss asked Waldman.

"George, I don't know," she said. "You're going to have to go there and find out."

After several telephone calls, he told her he would go, but only if there was no advance publicity for the show. The last thing he needed was every newspaper and television reporter in the New York metropolitan area camped outside the museum, ready to make a groveling spectacle of him.

Sworn to secrecy at the risk of abrupt cancellation, Waldman reached out to Berra through his son Dale and Dave Kaplan at the museum. When told of Steinbrenner's willingness to come, Berra reacted badly, seeing it as another gimmick. "The hell with it. He ain't coming here," he bristled.

Over the years, Berra had become almost deaf to those clamoring for him to make up with Steinbrenner and more partial to the people who applauded him for his principled stand. In 1998, for example, as the museum was preparing for its grand opening, Kaplan had received a call from *Sports Illustrated* requesting a photo shoot with Berra for inclusion in a piece the magazine was doing on "the greatest things in sports." Berra's stand against Steinbrenner had made the cut. Berra adamantly refused, on the grounds that his absence from the stadium spoke for itself.

He was also wary of the public nature of Waldman's proposal: a live radio show had all the trappings of a typical Steinbrenner promotion. That would put the meeting more on Steinbrenner's terms, even if on Berra's turf.

But Dale Berra was certain that on some level, his father always knew that the time had to come to stop refusing to so much as enunciate Steinbrenner's name. The owner of the Yankees couldn't forever be "that guy."

"Fourteen years is long enough, the most you can get out of it," Dale said, reminding Yogi of how difficult it would be for Steinbrenner to repent in the way Waldman was proposing.

Finally, when Dale sensed that his father was weakening, he played his ace, a personal plea from him and his brothers. "None of your grandchildren have ever seen you in the place you became so famous," he said. "Why continue to deny them?"

It wasn't entirely true that none of Berra's grandchildren had ever seen number 8 in pinstripes. Lindsay Berra, daughter of Larry, remembered Yogi in uniform in the early to middle 1980s, before the firing. Her grandmother would take her to the stadium, bringing along a basket of fried chicken because she knew how much Lindsay hated hot dogs.

When Lindsay was in high school, a friend invited her to a Yankees game. A sports lover and Yankees fan, she desperately wanted to go but felt she needed her father's permission. Although she had seen her grandfather watching games in his den — seated in his blue leather chair, pulling for the Yankees — she worried about offending him.

"Of course you can go," her father said, reminding her that Yogi's feud was with George, not the team. He still loved the Yankees; all the Berras did.

But by late 1998, the younger grandchildren having come of age, Dale's argument finally penetrated his father's defenses. Berra loved the children, all nine of them at the time, and relished having them in the Montclair area. "The kids were pretty strong on this," he said. "They said I had to give it a chance. I finally said OK, but I didn't know what the heck to expect. All I know is, Carmen had to be there; that I insisted on. Whatever George had to say, he had to say it to her, too."

Through the years, Steinbrenner believed it was Carmen who had been the most committed to the boycott—a mischaracterization of her and an underestimation of her husband's resolve. Yogi wanted Carmen with him because in his mind, they were a team. They both had suffered and sacrificed as partners in love and war. (Asked once by broadcaster Michael Kay which person he would most want to have in a foxhole with him, a question naturally aimed at getting him to reveal his most trusted teammate, Berra said, without hesitation, "Carmen.")

So the stage and the show were finally set, the big meeting to coincide with the December museum debut. And then, a couple of days before, Steinbrenner called Waldman to say he couldn't come. Tragedy had struck the Florida governor's mansion, where Lawton Chiles had collapsed during a workout and died of heart failure. As a well-known Florida businessman and owner of America's most famous sports team, Steinbrenner said that he was obligated to attend the governor's funeral, which unfortunately was scheduled for the day they had planned the show with Yogi. It would be impossible for him to reach New Jersey in time.

"Don't worry, I'll call Yogi," he promised.

Waldman chuckled. *Typical George,* she thought. In his mind, he believed he had made things right merely by agreeing to do the show; he and Berra were already on amicable terms.

"That's all right," she told him. "I'll take care of it. We'll reschedule."

She called WFAN with the news and then called Kaplan to postpone the big event. Her producer notified the handful of special guests she had lined up and booked them for the new date: January 5 of the brand-new year, a historic night that would reroute Berra's storybook life and the off-field narrative of Steinbrenner's Yankees.

Waldman could feel her pulse racing and beads of sweat forming a mosaic on her forehead when the door to Kaplan's office closed and a muffled but clearly raised voice came from inside. The men of the moment, the Boss and Yogi, had been ushered into the office after Steinbrenner had arrived at the museum.

Now Waldman was overwhelmed with fear and regret: Berra wasn't going to receive Steinbrenner graciously, or Steinbrenner wasn't going to show proper remorse, and all hell was going to break loose. Steinbrenner's humiliation would be blamed on her, and her countless hours of making herself an indispensable asset to WFAN would evaporate in the time it had once taken Mel Allen to marvel, on Yankees broadcasts, "How about that?"

Then Carmen Berra marched into Kaplan's office, while Waldman positioned herself behind a pole, unconsciously hiding in the event Steinbrenner stormed out. Bad as that would have been for her, she knew it would have been worse for him.

"Everyone else was concerned for Yogi, but my loyalties were with George," Waldman said. "The last thing that I wanted to see happen was for him to be embarrassed."

Twelve years after the fact, she recalled that the shouting had ceased with Carmen's entry. Had Waldman only imagined the raised voice? Or had it merely been a result of Steinbrenner's exuberance? Everyone could see he'd been a bundle of nerves.

No one who was in the room — the Berras or Steinbrenner — would remember any harsh words. Carmen recalled that Steinbrenner held Yogi by the shoulders, looked him in the eye, and said, "I know I made a mistake by not letting you go personally. It's the worst mistake I ever made in baseball."

Not given to long speeches, Berra replied, "I made a lot of mistakes in baseball, too."

They shook hands and emerged from the office. Carmen opened a bottle of champagne. They toasted new beginnings, and Berra proceeded to give Steinbrenner a tour of his new digs.

Two reporters, one from the *New York Times* and the other from the *Daily News* — Montclair residents who had been tipped off about the event by Kaplan—quickly corralled Berra and Steinbrenner for quotes before rushing off to make deadline with the news that the long feud was over.

Asked if his boycott of Yankee Stadium would end immediately, Berra was playfully noncommittal. "I told him what he needed to do," Berra said. "He apologized. We'll see."

For his part, Steinbrenner was deferential. "If I could get Yogi to come back," he said, "I'd bring him over with a rickshaw across the George Washington Bridge."

During the museum tour, a videographer working for the museum cornered Steinbrenner and asked for his take on Berra. The Boss, relaxed now, laid it on with classic Steinbrenner hyperbole.

"There have been great Yankees, and Yogi is right there at the top of that list," he gushed. "But there's probably never been a Yankee who heard more times, 'You can't do that; you can't do that,' and then just turned around and did it. Oh, he was a warrior, a warrior in every sense of the word, and you know how much I love that word. If I was in the trench, I'd want Yogi Berra with me."

If the feelings weren't mutual—Berra having already chosen Carmen for his trench-mate—he clearly enjoyed himself as he led Steinbrenner around the museum. Warming to the occasion, he praised Joe Torre and the Yankees staff and told Steinbrenner not to interfere, or he definitely wouldn't show up for another fourteen years.

When they stopped in front of a blowup of Berra throwing away his catcher's mask in front of home plate in a World Series game against the Brooklyn Dodgers, Berra explained to Steinbrenner the art of catching a knuckleball. By an old photo of the legendary Joe DiMaggio, Lou Gehrig, and Tommy Henrich, Steinbrenner told Berra how Henrich's restaurant in Columbus, Ohio, had been turned into the first Wendy's franchise.

Near a display for Larry Doby, another Montclair resident and Hall of Famer, Steinbrenner told Berra how much he admired Doby, who broke the American League color line in Cleveland, Steinbrenner's hometown.

Soon they moved into the museum's theater, with its replica scoreboard from the original Yankee Stadium and seating that looked like a section of the grandstand. Perched between Steinbrenner and Berra, Waldman began the show by announcing to her audience that something very special was about to happen.

She introduced her guests with a flourish: "Mr. Steinbrenner, you know Mr. Berra; Mr. Berra, Mr. Steinbrenner." There were smiles all around. Anxiety had given way to festivity.

At the outset of the show, the theater was empty except for the few invited guests. But as it proceeded, with Waldman fielding calls from Joe Garagiola, Berra's boyhood pal from St. Louis, and the great Ted Williams, word spread — something wonderful was happening at the museum — and people began arriving: men in their suits, fathers and sons, students from campus.

Less than an hour into the show, Waldman looked up from her microphone and was amazed to see that the theater was full. "They heard us," she said. "They heard that George Steinbrenner and Yogi Berra were making up, and they wanted to see it for themselves."

Berra especially got a kick out of Ted Williams's call. "Teddy Ballgame" — now that was about as big as it got in baseball. Berra told Steinbrenner that he was going to be inducted into Williams's museum in Hernando, Florida, the following month. Out of the blue, Berra asked Steinbrenner if he would attend the ceremony. Steinbrenner looked as if he might cry. The color had also returned to his face.

When the show was finished, the Boss gave Carmen a hug and told her, "He's got to forgive me and come back." She told Steinbrenner he had done the right thing by coming; she doubted there would be a problem anymore.

As Steinbrenner and Cerrone made their way to the back door, accompanied by Carmen and Yogi, the Boss clutched a copy of Berra's new book of original Yogi-isms and a museum T-shirt.

"Thank you for inviting me, Yogi," Steinbrenner said. "I'll talk to you soon."

The door closed behind Berra. He turned back with a smile that could have lit a blacked-out city.

"Fourteen years," he said. "It's over."

Cerrone had never seen Steinbrenner less restless, more at peace, than on the ride back to the city that night. "Like a cinder block had been lifted from his shoulders," he said.

Berra admitted that it had taken a brave man to come and apologize, especially when Steinbrenner knew that Berra "could be a rock head."

When Waldman called Steinbrenner that night to thank him, he was exhausted from the stress of the affair but said, "This was a very good day for the Yankees." Seldom at a loss for what served the interests of the media, he teased Waldman: "And a pretty good day for you, too."

Having long used Steinbrenner and the Yankees to boost circulation, the New York newspapers had a hot story for the next morning. The nascent reconciliation was front-page news in the *New York Times*. Both the tabloid *Post* and *Daily News* also blared, somewhat predictably, "It's Over."

The wit and wisdom of Yogi Berra was back in season.

4

Perfection

Ron Guidry was right where he had to be, in front of a television screen. It was early Sunday afternoon, July 18, 1999, the rare occasion when he wasn't about to miss the beginning of a weekend ballgame.

As much as he loved the Yankees and baseball, in that order, Guidry hated to waste a sunny, sultry Louisiana day lounging indoors. As an avid outdoorsman, he could never manufacture enough chores to do on his tractor around his sprawling property. For a few years, he ran baseball clinics for local children on a small diamond he had carved out of his own land — until it dawned on him that too many of the kids were there only because their parents wanted them to be and not because they actually loved to play baseball.

But whatever he was doing outside, Guidry would inevitably poke his head in the house, check the score with Bonnie, and time his return for the last half-hour or so of the game.

"I was always doing something throughout the day, staying busy," he said, punctuating each sentence, as he often did, by making good use of the plastic cup that served as his spittoon. "Bonnie has probably watched more games than I have," he added. "She'll be in the house, the TV on, and then I'll come back in, and we'll watch the end together."

That, of course, was subject to change once the playoffs commenced, when the intensity level rose to a kick-the-coffee-table level and the plaintive cries of *"Jesus Christ!"* would send his wife scurrying to watch in another room.

"She doesn't get nervous in the same way as me," he admitted. "Only when something bad happens to the pitcher, and then it's always somebody else's fault. Then she gets irate because it's charged to the pitcher."

Such was the life of a former pitcher's wife. Guidry, by contrast, only cared about which team in the end got the W. "I get upset because I get a feeling of what should be done, and I worry that the guy's not going to do it and the outcome's going to be horrible," he said.

July 18, 1999, wasn't supposed to be about the outcome or anything that happened in the game — at least not when 41,930 fans filed into Yankee Stadium for an interleague affair against the lowly Montreal Expos. That day, the main attraction was Yogi Berra. Yogi had already had the honor of throwing out the first pitch on Opening Day, but now he was back for his own special day to commemorate his return to the fold.

The Yankees had been promoting the event for weeks, plastering the newspapers with ads showing the 1984 *Sports Illustrated* photo taken from behind. This time, the implication was that Berra was back and wasn't going anywhere for a long, long time.

A decade into blissful retirement, Guidry still felt like part of the Yankees as well, given his spring training duties, his regular participation in Old-Timers' Day, and his lifelong habit of watching the Yankees on television from the comfort of his couch a few thousand miles away.

Thankfully for Guidry, the world had come a long way from when he and his mother had relished the few regular-season games televised nationally and when he had dashed home from school — like any New York City kid — to catch the last few innings of a weekday World Series game. By 1999, his almighty satellite dish was pulling in most Yankees games telecast on the MSG (Madison Square Garden) Network or WPIX (channel 11) in New York.

Best invention ever, as far as Guidry was concerned. Southwestern Louisiana might as well have been the north Jersey suburbs.

Just like Berra, Guidry had welcomed the birth of the Torre/Jeter era, watching on television as the Yankees won it all in 1996 for the first time since Guidry's dream season of 1978. After losing to Cleveland in the American League Division Series the following year, they played at a torrid pace in 1998, claiming 114 regular-season victories, followed by 11 more in the postseason, and sweeping the San Diego Padres in the World Series.

Yes, it was great to be a Yankee again, and especially today, Yogi Berra Day at Yankee Stadium. Guidry settled onto the couch with a cold drink in his hand and Bonnie alongside him. He remarked that the speech alone — if what Berra was about to give could be classified as such — might be the best thing he would see all season.

He had no idea.

In New York City, the day was steaming hot, destined to reach a high of 98 degrees, as a languid mass of humid air that might have been transported from the Louisiana bayous settled over the Bronx. But Berra stayed cool, taking part in a fundraising promotion for his new museum. For the trip from New Jersey to the famous ballpark, he and his family shared a New York Waterway boat with ticket-buying fans. Along the way, they detoured to a Manhattan dock to take aboard the Yankees-loving mayor of New York City, Rudy Giuliani. The mayor had grown up in Brooklyn and Garden City, an Italian boy who especially idolized Berra.

Joining Yogi were Carmen, their three sons, their grandchildren, and Yogi's only surviving sibling — his sister, Josie, who still lived in the same brick bungalow in the blue-collar neighborhood that Berra had grown up in. It was hard to believe that after so many years, she had never before stepped foot in Yankee Stadium. In effect, this was the day Dale Berra had sold to his father the previous winter when he had pleaded Steinbrenner's case.

When the "Good Ship Berra" reached the South Bronx shrine, the heavy air was laden with nostalgia and karma, beginning with the co-incidental fact that it was Joe Torre's fifty-ninth birthday. Then there was the always welcome sight of a certain former Berra battery mate.

Rather than have him reenact the Opening Day ceremony of throwing out the first pitch, the Yankees decided to have Berra take up his more natural position at home plate and catch it. In what would turn out to be a ceremonial stroke of genius, the Yankees flew Don Larsen in from his home in San Diego to re-create the perfect-game battery from game five of the 1956 World Series.

Also on the guest list were Berra's pals Joe Garagiola, Phil Rizzuto, Whitey Ford, Bobby Richardson, and Gil McDougald. For the occasion, a large number 8 was painted on the grass behind the plate. Berra rode onto the field and into view of the fans in a cream-colored 1957 Thunderbird convertible. Circling the dirt track around the field, Berra waved to the crowd as Louis Armstrong's "What a Wonderful World" blasted through the loudspeakers.

From the dugout, where she was providing broadcast updates, Suzyn Waldman looked on in tears, thinking, *I helped do this.* She was also mindful that she had done it not only for Berra but also for her friend, the Boss.

In the Yankees bullpen, David Cone warmed up for the start but was distracted by the sudden eruption of cheers. "I'd never had a warm-up like that, so happy-go-lucky, carefree," he recalled. "I wasn't even concentrating on my pitches, just watching Yogi riding around, laughing and waving at him when he came around the warning track. I had this tremendous feeling of being part of the Yankees family, of the tradition."

Cone knew Berra only in the way most players who had never dressed in the same clubhouse knew him. They went out of their way to meet him. As a member of the late-1980s Mets, Cone had walked across the field to introduce himself one day in Houston when Berra was coaching for the Astros. "If you've grown up loving and playing baseball and you see Yogi Berra on the field, how could you not?" Cone said.

Back at home plate, basking and broiling in the oppressive sun, broadcaster Michael Kay was already perspiring heavily in his suit as he prepared to emcee the ceremony, getting goose bumps himself when Berra stepped out of the Thunderbird. Kay was thinking he was in for one of the great day-night doubleheaders of all time, courtesy of a couple of Jersey icons: Berra and Bruce Springsteen, in concert that night across the river at the Continental Airlines Arena.

To begin, Derek Jeter — who at twenty-five was already the on-field face of the Yankees — presented Carmen Berra with a bouquet of flowers. Then it was Yogi's turn.

Forty years earlier, in 1959, a very different Yankees organization had staged the first Yogi Berra Day, highlighted by a presentation of fishing equipment by Ted Williams. Steinbrenner made sure that this one would be different. Berra received replicas of his ten championship rings, a trip to Italy for Carmen and him, a $100,000 donation to his museum, and the original 1951 championship banner — the third of five straight Yankees championships, coinciding with Berra's first MVP season.

Predictably, Berra's speech lasted about as long as it took for a young greyhound like Jeter to run out a slow ground ball. "I knew I'd get emotional talking," said Berra, who generally tried to avoid public displays of emotion. "I had to keep it short and thank the fans."

Naturally, he created a Yogi-ism for the occasion, thanking everyone for making him feel at home, because Yankee Stadium to him was home. "You're great," he told the fans, who responded by chanting his name.

Finally, the Yankees took the field, and it was time for Larsen and Berra to do their thing. Cone was at the mound, next to Larsen, waiting for Berra and the Yankees' starting catcher, Joe Girardi, to get their act together. Having never met Larsen, Cone made small talk, inquiring, "Are you going to jump into Yogi's arms again?"

Larsen laughed. "Kid, you got it wrong," he said. "He jumped into *my* arms." Cone stood corrected, making a mental note of how casually Larsen made the point, like a droll old-time Hollywood actor.

Meanwhile, Berra and Girardi were about to walk to the plate. "I remember in the clubhouse how excited everyone was about the day, that we were all going to be part of Yogi's day," Girardi said. He had already caught the first pitch Berra had floated to the plate on Opening Day — when Cone was also the Yankees' starter — and had rushed to the mound to hand him the ball, saying, "This is a great thrill." But now that Girardi was sharing the actual catcher's space with Berra, he felt as if he had stepped into a history book.

He remembered the smaller glove — about the size of the mitt Berra had used back in the day — he had occasionally trained with and had stored away inside the clubhouse. "You want me to go get the little glove for you, Yogi?" Girardi asked, figuring the prop might be nice for the throwback nature of the occasion.

"No," Berra told him. "I want to use yours."

Girardi handed it to him, making one ambitious request: "Put a blessing on it," he said.

When the Yankees scored five runs off the Expos' Javier Vázquez in the second inning — home runs by Derek Jeter and Ricky Ledee doing most of the damage — the suspense seemingly drained from the day. After Cone struck out the side in the top of the third, the skies darkened, and a thunderstorm briefly threatened to end the game before it was official.

Cone was thirty-six — the number he happened to wear on the back of his jersey. At that age especially, there was the risk that his shoulder would tighten up during the rain delay, particularly with the Yankees due to bat first when the game resumed. But then came an assist from Mother Nature. Not long after the thirty-three-minute delay, the sun was back out, and it was hotter and more humid than before, helping Cone to stay loose.

In fact, when he took the mound for the top of the fourth — having set down all nine hitters up to that point — he felt stronger than when he had started the game. His velocity — though not comparable to that in his more youthful days with the Mets — actually improved as the game progressed. With pinpoint control of his fastball and a biting slider, Cone had the Expos lunging all day, hitting weak flies to the outfield, if they made any contact at all.

None of what he had seen so far surprised Felipe Alou, the Expos' veteran manager. Alou had played with the Yankees during the early 1970s, when the franchise was in disarray under the sorry ownership of CBS and about to be sold to Steinbrenner. He knew there was no team in baseball that staged big events like the Yankees. He understood what Yogi Berra Day represented and why it had to be held. And he worried that his young, inexperienced team would be distracted by the sight of all the Yankees legends.

From a tactical standpoint, what was worse was the lineup card Alou had walked to home plate prior to the game. Not one of his hitters had faced Cone before. He watched as the crafty right-hander befuddled them, one after another, and felt helpless to do anything about it.

Having decided to watch the game with his large family, Berra looked on from suite 332. Meanwhile, Larsen watched from Steinbrenner's private box. As it turned out, they were the only invited guests who didn't pick up and leave after a few innings.

"There were plans to leave early, but I told everyone, 'I'm staying, you can go,'" Berra said. "After the fifth, I wasn't going anywhere." In the box with her grandparents and other relatives, Berra's granddaughter Lindsay sent her boyfriend on his way. He had a flight to catch to North Carolina. "You're on your own," she told him.

Walk out on a perfect game? A Berra wouldn't think of it. Even with four innings to go, and the odds stacked against Cone making it last into the ninth, Yogi was steadfast. There was, after all, some precedent for grand things happening in this ballpark. It had only been a little over a year since David Wells had thrown a perfect game against the Minnesota Twins — the first in Yankee Stadium since Larsen's.

No, Berra wasn't going home just yet, not on this day, *his* day. He thought Cone "could use a little luck," and who else was more capable of providing it than the man most baseball people considered — with all due respect to the memory of Lou Gehrig — the luckiest man on the face of the earth?

Knowing from firsthand experience how difficult it was to get all the way to twenty-seven outs without a hit or a walk, Berra normally didn't entertain the possibility until at least the end of the seventh inning. "If you get by the seventh, then you start thinking about it," he said. "You only need six more outs."

Cone's mastery of the Expos only grew as the innings rolled by. Rare was the called ball, accounting for a mere twenty of the eighty-eight pitches he wound up throwing.

Could this really be happening? Down on the field, with the heat index rising, Girardi looked up at the zeros on the scoreboard in the eighth inning and hoped he wasn't hallucinating. "I remember saying to myself, 'You have got to be kidding me,'" he said. "What explanation could there have possibly been other than Yogi and Larsen had graced us with their presence?"

Cone, meanwhile, dismissed the thought of upstaging Berra's day. The more correct interpretation, dawning on him after the sixth inning, was that if he could somehow pull off the implausible feat, he would actually be enhancing it. "The feeling of history started to build as the game went along, and at one point I was almost overwhelmed, thinking, you know, Wow, *this* could happen on this of all days," he said.

Berra was hoping, even praying, while unavoidably dwelling on his own close calls over a baseball lifetime, including one that got away. Would he ever stop blaming himself for the no-hitter Bill Bevens almost threw for the Yankees in the 1947 World Series against the Dodgers?

Pinch-running with one out in the ninth inning, Al Gionfriddo took off for second. The rookie Berra threw high, giving Gionfriddo the stolen base. After an intentional walk to Pete Reiser, Cookie Lavagetto hit a game-winning double — the Dodgers' only hit off Bevens.

It was much easier to live with the memory of dropping Ted Williams's twisting pop foul with two outs in the ninth on September 28, 1951, handing the best pure hitter in baseball another opportunity to ruin Allie Reynolds's no-hit bid. Williams hit the next pitch in nearly the same spot. Berra held on. Is it a reach to say that an angel of fortune spared him the cruelty of fate and a rare moment of infamy?

Berra had watched Mickey Mantle save Larsen's gem with a running catch that ranked on his all-time list of greatest catches. Based on all his experience, he suspected that Cone was sooner or later also going to need an assist from at least one of his teammates.

That moment came with one out in the eighth inning, when Jose Vidro hit a grounder up the middle ticketed for center field. Vidro had been one of the few Expos hitters to get ahead of Cone in the count. Loath to surrender the perfect game on a walk, Cone decided to gamble and challenge Vidro, a line-drive hitter.

"I got the better part of the middle of the plate, and he hit it up the middle," Cone said. "I thought, *There it goes.*"

Because Vidro was a switch hitter batting left, Yankees second baseman Chuck Knoblauch needed to protect the hole between first and second. To make the play, he had to get the best jump possible. He did, making a backhanded grab, turning and planting his feet for the throw. Now came an even bigger challenge for Knoblauch, who that season had developed a hitch in his throwing motion, a debilitating handicap that would soon require a shift to the outfield.

With the speedy Vidro dashing toward the bag, Knoblauch had no time to think, only to react. Somehow, he held it together, defied the psychological demons, and kept it simple, Berra-style. He fired a strike to Tino Martinez at first for the twenty-third out.

Berra was beside himself now, more nervous watching a ballgame than he had been in years. In the ninth inning, Cone fanned Chris Widger on three pitches for his tenth strikeout of the game. Ryan McGuire, a left-handed hitter, pinch-hit for the right-handed Shane Andrews. He lofted a lazy fly ball into short left field.

On came Ledee, circling a little too tentatively. Cone worried that he hadn't picked it up in the late afternoon haze. Berra, who had endured his share of unsteady moments in the same Yankee Stadium sun field, also could see that Ledee wasn't sure of himself.

He made the catch, using two hands. Berra exhaled. "When the kid caught the ball in the sun after not seeing it, I thought that could be the break," he said.

The twenty-seventh and last batter, shortstop Orlando Cabrera, swung at the first pitch and missed. He took the second for a ball. Then Cone unleashed a fastball, and Cabrera popped it up behind third. Cone's hands were already on the top of his cap, a sign of disbelief, as he watched the ball settle into Scott Brosius's glove.

In an instant, the weight of his achievement dropped him to his knees and onto the grass in front of the mound. Here came Girardi, wrapping Cone up before the others piled on, just like Berra and Larsen. Up in Steinbrenner's box, the tears Berra had managed to stave off during the pregame festivities now rolled down his cheeks.

He rode the elevator down to the clubhouse with Larsen, stopping in Torre's office to say, "My day and Don Larsen's here, this was great." Then they went to congratulate the man of the hour. They took plenty of photos, Cone wanting to make sure he had every base covered for his own collection and posterity.

On the day the Yankees were honoring number 8, with the number painted on the grass behind the plate, Cone learned that he had delivered exactly 88 pitches to Girardi. "It was kind of like a miracle," he said later.

Cone would go 2–5 for the rest of that season, 4–14 the next. He came to believe that as a largely spent former all-star, he had been inspired by Berra to turn back the clock. Nor was it lost on Cone that

Larsen had been a marginal major-league pitcher, 81–91 over four-teen seasons. In the twilight of his own career, Cone had become Don Larsen.

While they celebrated in the clubhouse, Cone introduced Larsen to his marketing agent, Andrew Levy. Fresh in the pantheon of all-time Yankees performances, Cone told Larsen that perhaps Levy could help him out, assuming that Larsen had never really cashed in on his perfect game, at least by contemporary marketing standards. Cone was right; the extent of Larsen's "haul" over the years had been a few measly dollars per autograph.

In no time, a new business partnership was born. Levy signed Larsen as a client, increasing his bookings and teaming him up with Cone on occasion. And when the new Yankee Stadium opened in 2009, Levy purchased a private sanctuary there in which to entertain his clients. He named it the Perfect Suite.

With his museum open for business, Berra found new pathways to Yankees lore. In November, he hosted Larsen, Cone, Girardi, and Jorge Posada — who had caught David Wells's 1998 perfect game against Minnesota — for a panel discussion in front of a theater every bit as jammed as it had been ten months earlier for Steinbrenner and Berra. Wells was unable to attend due to a case of gout, but all were present for the closing of the old Yankee Stadium in September 2008. A "perfect photo" hangs in Berra's museum.

Berra's return to the Yankees created a revival for him as well, including a spate of books by him and about him. The week be-fore Cone's perfect game, he had signed a two-year deal to join the advisory board of an online auction house specializing in collect-ibles — and that was apart from a website that his son Tim was about to launch to sell Berra merchandising, including Yogi-autographed stuffed toy bears for $450 apiece.

Some Berra keepsakes were not for sale and never would be. One of them was the prize photo Girardi left the museum with — of Yogi holding his daughter, Serena, who was just a couple of months old. Another was the mitt Berra had borrowed to catch the ceremonial toss from Larsen. Girardi asked Berra to sign it, and he took it home as a souvenir of what felt like a day of magic—even to Berra, who had already lived a baseball lifetime in what felt like his own fantasy kingdom.

On the way home from the game, Yogi kept repeating to Carmen, "Can you believe it—a perfect game on my day?" It *was* hard to believe. But whatever the explanation, it was the best gift the Yankees ever gave him.

Down in Lafayette, Guidry watched the ceremony, Larsen to Berra, and could see how much Yogi enjoyed the moment. The smile—he knew that Berra didn't waste many—gave his feelings away.

Guidry had been excited for his old mentor from the time he had flipped on ESPN to learn of George Steinbrenner's apology on that January night six months earlier. He couldn't help but laugh and say to himself, "Goddamn, that old son of a bitch beat the odds." Who else could have pulled off such a coup?

"For me, I already knew Yogi had integrity, but I think George found out just how much he had over those fourteen years," Guidry said. "I think he miscalculated Yogi. I think what he didn't understand was that Yogi was different from all the guys he had hired and fired, and that showed by the fact that George wound up going to meet Yogi at his place, not the other way around."

Talking about Berra brought a glint to Guidry's eyes, a conviction to his words. "If Yogi had never come back, I wouldn't have been disappointed in him, because he stood up for what he felt was right, and whether Yogi was at the stadium or not, he was the Yankees," he said. "He *is* the Yankees."

In Guidry's mind, that was never plainer than on Yogi Berra Day, when Guidry went back in the house and Bonnie practically screamed the moment he walked through the door that David Cone was *pitching a perfect game!* Guidry was disoriented at first—"He's *what?*"—but he was quickly riveted to the television, forgetting for the moment how the day at the stadium had begun.

Both he and Bonnie could barely contain themselves—he as a pitcher who understood the incredible pressure Cone had to be feeling, and she as a pitcher's wife ready to condemn the poor fielder who might blow the game for him.

When Brosius squeezed the last out, Guidry's first thought was that the outcome was as much about Berra as it was about anyone. It was a message from an authority much higher than the commissioner telling Steinbrenner and the world that he had done the right thing and here was his reward.

"You know, everybody always says that Yogi is lucky, but I don't think it is luck," Guidry said, nodding, affirming his own contention. "I think it's karma, and I'll tell you something else, and I honestly believe this: if he wasn't there, it wouldn't have happened. It just wouldn't have happened."

Not that Berra was much interested in taking credit, at least not any more than for what he could contribute as one man on a roster of many. For him, it was always about the team—and one team in particular. As such, July 18, 1999, could best be explained by the most famous threads in American sports.

"Those pinstripes," Berra said, "they make you do something."

5

Campers

George Steinbrenner owned a hotel. Ron Guidry had a truck. The transformation of a baseball mentorship into a forever friendship was launched on the itinerant details of spring training life.

In the early days of the Yankees' 2000 camp, Yogi Berra was due to touch down in Tampa to begin the next and most natural phase of his reconciliation with the team. While the previous season had presented endearing occasions — throwing out and catching first pitches, suiting up for Old-Timers' Day, and being introduced by the godlike intonations of Bob Sheppard — ritualistic formalities weren't what Berra had yearned for over the past fourteen years.

"My dad never felt like he wasn't a part of the Yankees and would never have wanted to go back to the stadium just for a standing ovation," Dale Berra said.

But not being around the guys, in the clubhouse, in uniform, now that was painful. That's what he missed.

And then Steinbrenner, still basking in the goodness of his gesture from the previous winter, called in early 2000 with another proposal for his new best friend. Go to spring training, the Boss implored. Get back on the field. "I want you to look at our catchers," he said.

The offer excited Berra to the point that it was all he could do not to run to the closet and pack a bag, months in advance. He suspected and hoped that his focus as a guest instructor or adviser or whatever the Yankees would call him would be on Jorge Posada, who had become the number one catcher and was slated to carry an even heavier burden with the departure of Joe Girardi to the Cubs.

Posada—a strong, switch-hitting onetime minor-league infielder—was still considered a work in progress. As a former catcher, Joe Torre had mentored him behind the plate, but a manager had a multitude of responsibilities and only so much time to devote to one player. Berra would get the chance to observe Posada's mechanics up close and personal over a period of a few weeks.

This would not be his first trip to the Yankees' complex in Tampa, where the team had relocated from Fort Lauderdale in 1996, eleven years into the Berra boycott. Weeks after Steinbrenner's apology in January 1999, he had dropped by for a day while in Florida with Carmen. He'd kibitzed with Derek Jeter and outfielder Bernie Williams, telling Williams he had never been able to play guitar because his fingers were too fat. He'd watched an intrasquad game while perched between Torre and bench coach Don Zimmer. He'd worn a Yankees cap that Torre had graciously placed on his head.

But his new assignment was different. It was special. It would put him in the clubhouse on a daily basis, back in full uniform, cap to cleats. He would watch exhibition games from the dugout. Finally, after fourteen years, he would be a Yankee *with* the Yankees.

As January surrendered to February, and as the traditional countdown to pitchers and catchers intensified, Berra couldn't wait to hit the road and to hear the familiar sounds of spring training—the banter in the clubhouse, the clomping of players on their way to the batting cages, the smack of ball making angry contact with glove.

All he needed was his plane ticket, his hotel reservation, and a ride to the hotel from the airport in Tampa. On the morning of his departure, he asked Joni Bronander, who handled event planning for his museum and who had had Guidry's DRIVING MR. YOGI cap custom-made, if a limousine would be waiting for him.

As a matter of fact, she said, Ron Guidry called and said that he will be there to get you.

"Gator?" he asked.

Yes, Bronander said. *That* Ron Guidry.

"When we found out that he was coming, everybody started looking forward to it," Guidry said. "I mean, we're not talking about John Doe here; we're talking about Yogi Berra."

He had heard that morning of Berra's impending arrival in the afternoon and thought it would be nice if someone Berra actually knew showed up to greet him, as opposed to an anonymous driver. Berra, after all, was now by consensus proclamation "the Greatest Living Yankee" following the death of Joe DiMaggio the previous year, but Berra didn't exactly welcome the moniker.

"What about Whitey and Phil?" he said when the subject came up, referring to his pals Ford and Rizzuto. "They're pretty good, you know."

Berra was the opposite of DiMaggio, who wore the appellation like the most ostentatious bling and demanded reverence from everyone within a two-hundred-mile radius. When the Yankees dared introduce Mickey Mantle after him during one Old-Timers' Day — to spare DiMaggio the wait through prolonged applause for the recently retired Mick — Joe D. wailed as if they had moved his monument into the men's room.

When Guidry played, he liked to observe the old-timers as they got reacquainted and mingled in the clubhouse. "When Joe D. and Yogi were both there, he had more people talking to him than there were talking to Joe D., I can tell you that," Guidry said.

Berra was an entirely different breed from DiMaggio, almost oblivious to the impact his return to spring training would have on the clubhouse. "We were all thrilled he was coming back and was going to be with us on a daily basis," said Joe Torre. "It felt like a special day, a holiday. We all wanted to do whatever we could to make him feel comfortable."

For a man of unyielding habit, Berra was facing adjustments of his own, having been away for so long. He didn't know his way around the complex, much less the Tampa area. The staff was unfamiliar, the broadcasters were different, and the players barely knew him.

At least Steinbrenner was still perched in his box. Torre and two of his coaches, Mel Stottlemyre and Don Zimmer, were baseball lifers with whom Berra was at ease. And the guest camp instructors were all players he had coached in the late seventies. If there was one commodity the Yankees never seemed to run short of, it was retired legends, certified champions, to remind their current stars of what had come before them. It was one of the sweetest parts of spring training, the old guard again in pinstripes.

In fact, Steinbrenner asked Guidry back before he'd stepped one foot out the door following his retirement press conference in July 1989. The Boss had never forgotten how Guidry, at the height of his success as a starting pitcher in 1979 and only three years after Steinbrenner himself had questioned his character, had volunteered to pitch out of the bullpen as the closer after Goose Gossage tore a ligament in the thumb of his pitching hand while roughhousing in the clubhouse with catcher Cliff Johnson. "First he's for the Yankees, second he's for Guidry," Steinbrenner had raved. "Would that every Yankee act like him."

For better or worse, Steinbrenner had a long memory when it came to his ballplayers. In Guidry's case, it was all for the better. After he finished his retirement press conference, he was handed a note from the Boss that read: "I'd like to see you in my office after the interviews." Guidry rode the elevator to the owner's lair, where Steinbrenner asked him a favor.

"What the hell could I possibly do for you?" Guidry said.

"I'd like you to continue to come to spring training," Steinbrenner said. "Be there for me, for the organization. Just walk around, look at the pitchers. One thing I know is that you'll say what you think, because you always have."

Guidry couldn't argue with Steinbrenner on that point. At age thirty-eight, with a career record of 170–91, he still believed he could help the Yankees on the mound and had told them as much. They had apparently disagreed, but he wasn't bitter. He had achieved everything he'd wanted to do in baseball. But he still felt like a Yankee, and the commitment to Steinbrenner would only take him away from Lafayette for a few weeks. What the hell, he told the Boss. Sure, he'd go to spring training.

The following February and for every February after that, with the exception of the strike year, 1995, he'd made the familiar drive to Tampa, put on number 49, and gone to work for managers — Dallas Green, Bucky Dent, Stump Merrill, Buck Showalter — who came and went with a mind-numbing frequency while the franchise tried to pull itself together.

By 2000, with Torre entrenched as the paternal face of New York sports, the Yankees were a far more stable and successful organization than the one Guidry had left. They had three championships in four years, and they had a revered nucleus of players that reminded him of his late-seventies group. True, the Bronx was no longer burning, and no one confused the clubhouse with the borough's famed zoo. But Torre's Yankees had just as much competitive zeal and professional commitment as Billy Martin's, with far fewer headaches.

If Guidry could still revel in dressing next to former teammates such as Goose Gossage, Graig Nettles, and Mickey Rivers, there was also an inescapable ache in his heart that spring. The previous fall, weeks before the Yankees' sweep of the Atlanta Braves in the World Series, they had lost yet another iconic member of the extended family when Catfish Hunter had died of complications related to ALS, also known as Lou Gehrig's disease.

Guidry loved the like-minded Hunter — a no-nonsense strike thrower and incorrigible wisecracking country boy from North Carolina. He knew how much bodily dysfunction and pain Hunter had endured in the years after he was stricken. His death was still shattering, in some ways as difficult to fathom as Thurman Munson's tragic plane crash in 1979.

Berra was also hurt by Hunter's passing. He had admired the pitcher's tenacity and his straightforward demeanor. But even on the subject of death, Berra could charm the melancholy out of anyone, just as he had Whitey Ford at one Old-Timers' Day. Turning to his old pal while the list of that year's deceased scrolled down the scoreboard, Berra had confided, "Boy, I hope I never see my name up there."

Berra had a reservation to stay at Steinbrenner's hotel, the Bay Harbor Inn, in the Westshore district of Tampa, a few minutes' drive from the airport and the Yankees' complex. Guidry just happened to be lodging at an apartment complex right down the road. He didn't like staying in hotels, preferring to have a kitchen where he could prepare and enjoy a home-cooked meal, especially when Bonnie came to visit. Little did he know that the situational arrangement — meaning his proximity to Berra — would demand regular dining out, a routine that would become as much a part of spring training as pitchers and catchers.

"There was no real plan when he came in," Guidry said. "It just made sense [for me to pick him up at the airport], because I knew I'd be done at the ballpark by the time he landed and I was staying right there anyway."

Berra was thrilled to see Guidry and, as always, couldn't help but marvel at how he managed to look more in shape than many of the active players.

"What are you doing here?" he asked.

"No, what are *you* doing here?" Guidry replied, already tweaking Berra for abandoning his boycott.

Berra appreciated Guidry's wry sense of humor. They had a good laugh and shook hands. Guidry loaded Berra's bags into his truck, drove Berra to the hotel, and helped him inside. But he sensed that Berra was a bit uneasy, a little unsure of himself.

When Berra remarked that he hadn't packed certain items that he would need, toiletries and the like, Guidry suggested that they go shopping.

"What are you doing for supper?" Guidry said on the way back.

Berra shrugged. It had occurred to Guidry that fourteen years was a long time to be away from spring training. In 1985, over in Fort Lauderdale, where the Yankees used to train, Berra would have had his routines, his favorite places to eat, his coaches and a staff member or two to keep him company.

"Well, we got a good place right over there," Guidry said, referring to a Caribbean restaurant called the Bahama Breeze across the street.

Hungry following his trip, Berra liked that idea. They made a date for dinner that would, in essence, never end.

"There was really nobody else that he had to sit and talk with, to be around after the day at the ballpark," Guidry said. "I knew that, so I just told him, 'I'll pick you up, we'll go out to supper,' and that's how it started."

Berra had worn three major-league uniforms in his life — those of the Yankees, the Mets, and the Astros. But the pinstripes, he admitted, "always felt right." They always fit best and still did at age seventy-four.

Well, yes, he had to admit that they made the uniform "a little baggy" in deference to those parts of the body that cannot defy gravity. But Berra, who prided himself on working the treadmill, keeping off excess weight, was generally pleased with the sartorial statement he could still make wearing his famous number 8.

Most of all, Berra was thrilled to be back in the clubhouse, pulling up his uniform pants, taking his sweet time, watching the familiar morning scene of players, coaches, and reporters shuffling about. In the coaches' room, next door to Torre's office and across the hall from the players' sanctum, Berra felt pretty good about how the uniform would look on him when he finally stepped onto the field.

Unlike some other baseball septuagenarians he could name, such as the former Dodgers and Red Sox manager Don Zimmer, who was sitting nearby, sipping a cup of hot coffee. "What the hell happened to you?" he asked Zim, whose pinstripes surged well beyond his waistline.

But that first morning, despite savoring every step of the clubhouse routine, Berra didn't linger too long inside, anxious as he was to get a whiff of the manicured field. Uniform on, belt fastened, and cleats tied, he walked up the dugout steps, stepped onto the dirt track, and moved toward the batting cage. Among the fans out early to watch the morning workout — a good portion of them in Berra's age range, the loyal snowbirds — there were sounds of instant recognition. And suddenly there was a buzz in the crowd.

"It's not like the stands are full for a workout at that time of day," said Rick Cerrone, the media relations director at the time, who happened to be in front of the dugout when Berra walked out. "But we're the Yankees; people show up to see Jeter, Bernie Williams, and maybe the Boss. But all of a sudden, here comes number eight onto the field. You could hear the fans. It was if they were saying, *He's back! Yogi's back*. With all the popular players we had on that team, there was something magical about having Yogi walk out with us."

Berra the lovable ball buster was back, and he couldn't spend enough time around the park. With Guidry agreeing to sacrifice some sleep to get him to the park early, Berra was one of the first to arrive in the clubhouse every morning, and he quickly developed a routine.

He liked to hit the treadmill right away, so he could get in a workout before the players arrived. He didn't want to get in their way. Then it was on to the massage table to have Steve Donohue, the assistant trainer, work on his neck and shoulders. From there he would help himself to the telephone on Donohue's desk to call his guys around the country, Whitey and "Scooter" (Rizzuto) and Moose (Skowron), checking in like a gleeful kid reporting from sleepaway camp.

When Torre arrived, Berra would unfailingly join him in the manager's office for a breakfast of champions. With a history of family heart disease, Torre always watched what he ate, but he had become even more vigilant after being treated for prostate cancer in 1999. "Yogi would come in every morning and say, 'What are we having today — the egg whites, the oatmeal, the pancakes?'" Torre said.

After a low-fat feast, Berra worked the clubhouse and the complex, determined to develop relationships with the players who to that point he had mostly admired from afar, notwithstanding the games he had attended in 1999. He loved how fraternal they seemed. "Like the guys I played with," he said. "They don't fight. They just want to win."

From a distance, Guidry was amazed by the instant interaction, how quickly Berra and the players established a rapport. "They had a lot of veterans, guys from the eighties and nineties, throwback guys like David Cone, David Wells, Andy Pettitte, Scott Brosius," Guidry said. "They were a lot like the older guys who enjoyed the camaraderie. When Yogi first came back, he would sit in the clubhouse or on the bench, and they would come around him, include him in their everyday affairs. They would give him the respect he deserved. It wasn't just about them, the way it is now for a lot of the players."

When Berra interacted with them, Guidry gave him space, not wanting to intrude. He enjoyed watching Yogi work the room, thrilled not only by how the players were polite and welcoming but also by how much of a charge they seemed to get out of Berra. "And if you thought a lot of it was because he was just back, and it would have been enough to do it once or twice and then go about your business, it wasn't like that at all," Guidry said. "It was all spring. That's how he was treated. They were all around him every day, and he was around them."

Berra told Paul O'Neill how much O'Neill reminded him of Mickey Mantle, with his proclivity for taking out his frustrations on the water cooler or a wall. He took to calling Mariano Rivera "Skinny" and fascinated the best closer in baseball with tidbits about the earliest Latino ballplayers in the major leagues.

He never tired of reminding Derek Jeter of his team's failure to make the 1997 World Series. Had they won that series, Jeter's Yankees would have been challenging Berra's Yankees' record of five straight titles between 1949 and 1953.

When he wasn't chiding Jeter about collective achievements, he might rag on him about a personal failure. Once he stopped by to tell him that he had looked terrible striking out on a high 3–2 pitch the night before.

"Why did you swing at that?" Berra asked.

"Well, you swung at those pitches," Jeter replied.

Berra, the epitome of the bad-ball hitter, thought about that for a moment and snapped, "Well, I hit those; you don't."

A couple of nearby players cracked up, as did Jeter, who wasn't often the welcoming target of the needle. But few had the ability to wield a zinger as good-naturedly as Berra.

If there was one player in the 2000 camp who reminded Berra a bit of his free-swinging self, it was the young infielder from the Dominican Republic, Alfonso Soriano. Soriano's selectivity was almost nonexistent. While the Yankees loved his power, especially for an infielder, they were alarmed by his strikeout totals — 179 in 939 minor-league at bats.

Berra had prided himself on being a free swinger who wasn't a strikeout liability. Failing to put the ball in play was for him a source of embarrassment. In 1950, a season he did *not* win the MVP, he struck out 12 times in 597 at bats, an almost ludicrous figure for the kind of pitches he routinely attacked.

One day Berra took it upon himself to strike up a conversation with Soriano, who spoke passable English. They were soon joined by Torre, who told Soriano that Berra was probably the best bad-ball hitter in baseball history. Torre suggested to Berra that he might want to explain his philosophy to the kid. Berra was happy to oblige, and the result sounded something like the script of his Aflac commercial.

"Well, if you see it, hit it," he said. "Sometimes you don't see it. I'd let it go, and the next time I'd swing at it. I saw it better the next time."

Torre couldn't tell if Soriano had any idea what Berra was talking about. "But if you thought about what Yogi was saying, it made perfect sense," he said.

If Berra loved being around the players, the feeling was mutual. "The whole place lit up," David Cone said. "He just had that kind of energy. It's hard to explain, but he just garnered so much respect — though he never walked around commanding it. Guys would just want to talk to him, ask him questions, trying to get him to say one of his Yogi-isms.

"He loved the attention, loved talking baseball, and it felt like we had this good-luck charm, especially after the perfect game on his day. It gave all of us a sense of belonging, a sense of history, right in the middle of our little run. You know, here we were, trying to win three in a row, four out of five, and with Yogi there, it was sort of a confirmation. But it also kept us in check, because with as many rings as we had won, he was going to have more than twice that. A good notion to keep in mind: *Yeah, we're doing something special here, but look at what Yogi did.* You know, keep it in perspective."

Early on, Torre told Berra that he could participate as much or as little as he wanted to. He could take a day off when he felt like it, play a round of golf.

"Yog, you don't have to go with us for the night games," Torre said.

"What do you mean?" Berra complained. "I want to go."

Mostly, he was anxious to work with Jorge Posada, with whom he had chatted once or twice the previous season but didn't really know. Posada, a twenty-fourth-round draft pick, hailed from Puerto Rico but had attended community college in Alabama. He was bright, affable, and somewhat sensitive to criticism. At the same time, he was amazed that his personal tutor was Yogi Berra.

"I remember that spring training so well because we spent so much time together," he said. "Yogi was always with the catchers, going through the drills, blocking balls, watching us, laughing with us. It was amazing — you could tell how much he was enjoying it. I mean, we're thinking, *This is Yogi Berra. We should be honored to be in his presence*. But the way he acted, it almost was like it was the other way around.

"He made you feel that way. He was in uniform, first one out there every morning. He'd come out and say, 'It's too hot to block balls today, no blocking balls.' Or we'd have everyone out there — pitchers, infielders — and we'd be going through the drills, and all of a sudden he'd say, 'The catchers are done today; go home.' He didn't believe in overdoing it like some of the younger coaches. He was so much fun. He took care of us. Not every day but a few days. He understood what it was like to go through that stuff."

Berra worked with all the catchers in camp, but he watched Posada intently. During idle moments, he sat with Posada, telling stories of his early days as a struggling catcher.

"I was terrible," he said. "My throws sailed; my footwork was bad. The pitchers didn't like pitching to me."

"What changed?" Posada asked.

"Bill Dickey," he said, assuming Posada had heard of the Hall of Fame catcher and career-long Yankee. Dickey had come out of retirement in 1949 to tutor Berra — or, as Berra explained at the time, "to learn me his experience."

Dickey taught Berra tricks of the trade — how to handle foul balls and pop flies, block the plate, balance himself to throw out base stealers, and be the extension of the manager on the field. His mentorship helped Berra mature from a good-hitting catcher who was a liability behind the plate into a fellow Hall of Famer.

Now it was Berra's turn to pass along what Dickey had taught him. In a sense, he had also "unretired" to take on the job of making Posada *want* to catch, of making him believe he could contribute behind the plate as much as he could while standing alongside it with a bat in his hands. That is what Dickey had done for Berra, and he was eternally grateful.

"One thing I saw, Posada was overly concerned with the runners — he'd call too many fastballs," Berra said. "I told him his main responsibility was getting the hitter. I told him how to cheat when catching a breaking ball, move into the pitch. Too many guys don't do that too good."

Berra also advised Posada to know his pitchers — "which ones you can yell at, which ones you baby a bit. They're all different." He told Posada how he would take a few steps toward the mound and scream at Vic Raschi, "Come on, Onion Head, throw the damn ball." As time passed, he got a kick out of how hard-nosed Posada was with the Cuban right-hander Orlando "El Duque" Hernandez. It reminded him of his own obdurate approach with Raschi, who pitched better when he was mad.

Seeking to give Posada whatever edge he could, Berra asked him if he would consider trying a catcher's mitt similar to one Berra had used — featuring a fishnet webbing, which he always believed enabled him to see the pitched ball better and helped with squeezing foul tips. It was the kind of mitt he had used to catch Don Larsen's perfect game (later bronzed and put on display at the Yogi Berra Museum).

Posada was taken aback but flattered by Berra's offer. He gave Yogi one of his mitts, which Berra brought to a craftsman named John Golomb, who was known as "the Glove Doctor." Golomb replaced Posada's webbing with one similar to that in Berra's old mitt.

Posada gave it a try. He didn't feel comfortable but was reluctant to tell Berra for fear of hurting his feelings.

"I didn't care," Berra said. "The catcher's equipment has gotten a little different — it's all lightweight and fiberglass stuff."

Berra had no ego invested in the offer. It was just another idea to help Posada relax behind the plate. Better yet, it helped Posada build a sense of trust in Yogi. He could plainly see how much Berra wanted to make him a better catcher. And according to Posada, he succeeded.

"Having him right there, talking about what he thought we should do, keeping my hand closer to my glove, helped me a lot," Posada said. "But maybe the most important thing he helped me with was with his view of the game, knowing how hard it is but that you really needed to keep a positive attitude every day — that was very big for me. It wasn't like he gave long speeches. It was the little things he said, very simple things, but you never forget how many rings this guy has or that he's a Hall of Famer. Honestly, after a couple of weeks, it felt like he had been there forever."

In many ways, he had. Now everyone could see him and hear him and touch him. Berra quickly became the living link between championship generations, a man who early in his career had been photographed with the dying Babe Ruth and now was mentoring players in the twenty-first century.

Never one to overanalyze anything or rhapsodize about the glories of spring training, the essence of renewal, Berra allowed the players to contemplate the meaning of it all. Asked later how it had felt to be back, he said, "Sure, I was glad to be there. It was good being around everyone, Joe and all the coaches." He paused for a moment, then added, "Besides, it beat the cold back home."

Spring training, where repetition reigns, had always been the ideal environment for Berra. Long before he became one of baseball's grand elders, he was a man of time-honored routines, set in his ways. "If the doctor tells him to take a pill at nine A.M., the bottle is open at five of nine," Carmen Berra said.

But there was one Berra habit that Carmen always hated. That was his cigarette smoking and, worse, his fondness for chewing tobacco. Baseball players had forever been stuffing it into their cheeks, despite medical warnings, some gruesome cancer cases, and impassioned pleas to cease and desist from the likes of the outspoken Joe Garagiola, Berra's childhood friend and himself a reformed chewer.

Carmen convinced Yogi to stop smoking and chewing after he retired from baseball. He took up Dentyne gum as a substitute, especially as he aged and experienced cotton mouth from various medications. But back in the spring training environment, back with the guys, boys would be boys. And since Guidry was still a dedicated user of Skoal, a popular brand of chewing tobacco, and typically carried a small container in his back uniform pants pocket, Berra figured, what the heck, how much could a little bit before each game hurt? No more, he thought, than the three ounces of vodka he rewarded himself with every evening during dinner.

In his first spring back with the team, he developed one of his classic routines. On the bench as the game got under way, he would signal Guidry with a little nudge of the shoulder — his way of asking him to reach into his pocket, open the container, and hand him a small chew.

One day, when the game was being beamed back to New York on cable, the television camera happened to swing around to the dugout just as Guidry was handing Berra a wad that he packed into his cheek. Watching at home, knowing full well that Guidry wasn't handing Berra a stick of Dentyne, Carmen nearly jumped out of her seat. Later in the day, she was on the phone to her husband and Guidry, giving them both a piece of her mind. "After that," Guidry said, "I was always looking out for the cameras."

Guidry had never realized the extent of Berra's need for repetition and precision until that first spring training back, when Berra began peppering him with questions. In Berra-speak, he needed to know everything he didn't need to know.

"Like if he heard they had brought in a kid from the minor-league camp across the street and he wasn't on the roster list," Guidry said. "He needed to know the players, all of them. If he had the sheet with the names in his hand, well, he just saw a number seventy-two walk by in the clubhouse, so how come there's no seventy-two on the list? 'Yog, I don't know. They got twenty-five or thirty major-league guys in camp and another thirty or so young guys. You're not gonna know every single guy.'

"But he had to know *every single guy.* He'd say, 'I saw this tall kid yesterday. I watched him throw the other day, left-handed kid. I like him.' And I'd say, 'Which kid? Give me a name.' So he gives me the name, and I say, 'Yogi, he's right-handed.' And he says, 'No, not that kid. The left-handed kid.' I say, 'What's his name?' He says, 'I don't know. That's why they need to put the damn name on the list so I can tell him by the number.'"

Guidry quickly learned that lateness around Berra was not an option. When he offered Berra a ride to the complex after their first dinner out at the Bahama Breeze, he didn't quite realize that he had committed himself for the rest of the spring. "But once you did something, well, it had to be format, part of the regimen," he said. "When he does it one day, it's going to be that way for the next thousand days."

Berra could have rented a car, driven himself, but as he said, "Gator knew his way around. I couldn't tell you anything or anywhere. They had all these highways and traffic by the complex, a big change from Fort Lauderdale. Everything was real close in the old place."

Every morning, Guidry pulled up in his truck, typically a few minutes early in accordance with Berra Standard Time. Unfailingly, Berra was outside before Guidry rolled to a stop, often shaking an admirer's hand or having a photo snapped. But one morning, Guidry was delayed, pausing in the parking lot of his apartment complex to assist a damsel in distress.

"I had walked out about twenty minutes to seven to get into the truck," Guidry said. "There was a young lady a couple cars down from me. Her hood was up, [and] she was trying to start her car. It wouldn't start, so I asked her if I could give her a hand, see what it was. I got out my jumper cables, started my car, and got her going."

But now Guidry was ten minutes behind schedule and had two stop signs and a long red light to get through. He arrived at 7:02, two minutes late. As he did every morning, he rolled the truck to a stop right in front of the hotel, reached over and opened the door. Berra looked at him unhappily. "Where the hell you been?" he said.

"Yogi, you got grandchildren, right?" Guidry said.
Berra nodded.
"You got girl grandchildren?"
Berra nodded.
"Well, when I got to the truck, there was this young girl. She left

her lights on, her battery was dead, and I had to jump-start her car," Guidry said. "You're gonna be mad at me because I was helping her? She could have been your granddaughter, for Chrissakes."

Guidry couldn't figure out whether Berra's grumpiness about him being two minutes late was more exasperating or comical. Finally he blurted out, "Aw, just get your ass into the truck so we can go."

"OK, OK," Berra said, obediently climbing aboard with a shit-eating grin. Guidry looked at him and instantly realized that Berra actually liked being yelled at. Demanding as he could obviously be, he didn't want to be treated like some fragile family heirloom or icon.

"He doesn't want to be treated like royalty," Guidry said. "He wants to be picked on. So while I respected him and I wanted to do everything that I could for him, I decided that I wasn't going to let him get away with murder. I started to tease him all the time. I'd say, 'Look, the whole freaking world doesn't revolve around you. Son of a bitch, we got things we got to do.'"

That they did. And the ride was just beginning.

6

Shared Values

It made perfect sense to Ron Guidry that wherever he went with Yogi Berra in Tampa, Berra had admirers who seldom were shy about walking right up and saying, "Hello, how ya doing, would you mind signing this for my ailing brother in Topeka?" About town, Berra was more than a Hall of Fame catcher, a ten-time World Series winner, and an immortal Yankee. He was akin to a Disney character greeting visitors at the gates of his portable Magic Kingdom. Who, after all, would think twice about approaching a diminutive and elderly gentleman named Yogi?

But what did amaze Guidry was how Berra could be so remarkably unfazed by the fuss and equally unassuming about the need for it in the first place. On many a night out, dinner inevitably turned into a quasi–autograph session, with Guidry coming to the conclusion that Berra was "the most beloved man in America," and maybe the most tolerant.

Only once could he recall Berra losing patience with well-wishers, and that was at the Bonefish Grill on the bawdy commercial strip known as Dale Mabry Highway, a couple of miles from downtown Tampa.

"We were there for maybe the third or fourth time, and all of a sudden there was a huge crowd around the table," Guidry said. "He was besieged when he sat down to eat, and that he didn't like."

Berra didn't complain, though. He scrunched up his face just enough to let Guidry know that he felt as if the attention was an intrusion on their time together, their chance to live and breathe baseball, which was the whole point of spring training to begin with.

By then, Berra and Guidry had established an easy rapport and a five-restaurant rotation — the Bahama Breeze, the Rusty Pelican, Fleming's Prime Steakhouse, Lee Roy Selmon's, and the Bonefish. After several visits, when they called ahead for reservations, a staff member would greet them at the door and try to provide a table with the most privacy.

But after the incident at the Bonefish Grill, Berra wasn't keen on going back there. He liked the food, though, so when Tino Martinez mentioned another Bonefish Grill on Henderson Boulevard, approximately the same distance from the hotel, Berra said, "Good, we can go *there*." Replacing one franchise location in rotation with another was his idea of radical change.

Occasionally, he and Guidry brought along an invited guest — Don Zimmer, Steve Donohue, Goose Gossage, Stump Merrill, a visiting wife or child. The younger of Guidry's two daughters, Danielle, would visit for a few days most springs, and it didn't take long for her to develop a feisty rapport with Berra that tickled her father no end.

For Guidry, there also had to be time off for good behavior. He just couldn't eat out every night, sometimes aching for a burger and a beer in his apartment. "Stay in your damn room tonight; have a ham sandwich," he would say to Berra.

To which Yogi would respond, "OK, Gator. Where we goin' tomorrow?"

Guidry would laugh, flattered that Berra never took his mock repudiation personally or seriously.

If he had initially invited Berra to dinner out of a sense of obligation, noting that Yogi didn't have the social options he once had and especially without Carmen in town, Guidry was quick to add that never for a second did he consider the gesture charity or a chore. His respect for Berra and for what he meant to baseball and the Yankees was part of his childhood romance with the game, having grown up a fan of Berra's team.

It wasn't long before Guidry began looking forward to their nights out and realizing that if anyone was the beneficiary of the relationship, it was him. "I had this man who's a damn baseball history book, the perfect encyclopedia, sitting across the table from me, a guy who has seen everything," Guidry said.

The challenge was how to pry it open. Berra was not a loquacious man, speaking with the terseness of a text message before there was such a thing. As his son Dale liked to say, "He's the most quoted man in the world, and he never says anything."

But Guidry believed it wasn't how much Berra had to say; it was *what* he had to say and how much his companion wanted to hear it. "It was like when I played, you have to ask him things," Guidry said. "Just because he's old, that doesn't mean he doesn't remember. He doesn't just come out with it. You have to reach out and touch him, and then you'll be surprised by what happens. So we're sitting at the table and it's, 'Hey, tell me about the time you did this and that, tell me about this guy or that guy.'"

Tell me about Mickey Mantle and Roger Maris and the famous home run chase of 1961.

"I always wanted to know about Whitey Ford, Mickey Mantle, Roger Maris, because at that time, that's the early sixties, I'm a teenager, I'm pretty much deep into everything, and not only am I playing, but I understand more about it," Guidry said. "And I understand about all those guys that were playing. Years later, when I got to the Yankees, I'd see them all at an old-timers' game, but I didn't bother them too much, asking about those things you'd really want to know. That wasn't my thing."

He was, in other words, like any other young man who comes face-to-face with his boyhood idols. "It took me a whole bunch of years before I even shook Maris's hand," he said. "I was so afraid to talk. He was the only guy I wanted to say hello to that I never had the courage to, because, you know, with all the past things I had heard, how private a man he was."

Ever the social conduit, Mantle intervened in the clubhouse early one Old-Timers' Day. He and Ford were chatting, while Maris sat by himself two or three dressing stalls away. Guidry was sitting nearby.

"Ron," Mantle said, "have you met Roger?"

"No, but I'd like to," Guidry said.

Mantle called out to Maris, "Hey, Rog, you ever meet Guidry here?"

Maris looked up with a welcoming smile. "No, I've been dying to, though," he said.

Guidry stood up, shook Maris's hand, and berated himself for waiting so long. He never saw Maris at an Old-Timers' Day again. Maris died the next year, 1985, at the age of fifty-one.

"You say to yourself, 'You're such an idiot, you could've been talking to this man for years and years, and now all of a sudden . . .'"

Guidry had always wondered about the relationship between Mantle and Maris. He had heard conflicting stories about when they went head-to-head for the home run record, chasing Babe Ruth. Was it true that they were close enough friends that Mantle actually moved into Maris's apartment in Queens? He asked Berra how two so very different men could have lived together under such daily pressure.

"Nah, it wasn't like that," Berra said. "Mickey would go over and stay with Roger for a couple of days, and Roger would cook, Mickey would eat. Roger was just trying to get Mickey to stay in a little more because of what he meant to the club going down the stretch and in the World Series. They had their moments, but it wasn't like he moved in."

Guidry asked about the toll the pursuit took on Maris — the overwhelming sentiment for Mantle, the resentment of Maris for having the audacity to try to beat Babe Ruth's record.

"Oh, yeah, it was tough on Roger," Berra said, describing the late-season game in Baltimore when the Orioles brought in the masterful knuckleballer Hoyt Wilhelm just to keep Maris from hitting his sixtieth home run in the Yankees' 154th game, the same point in the season when Ruth had hit his.

"We were all mad," Berra said. "You know, the wind was blowing in, and they bring in a knuckleballer to make sure he didn't get it. We were all hollerin' over at them about that."

Berra told Guidry that what happened with Maris—the abuse he took, mainly from the defenders of Ruth, reporters and fans, and even the commissioner—was one of the saddest episodes he had seen in the game.

"He actually did lose his hair, and Roger was never the same after that," Berra said. In retrospect, Guidry felt better about not having brought the subject up with Maris, but his compassion for the man grew exponentially.

A good deal of what Berra told Guidry was in the history books, or probably in a book that Berra himself had published. But hearing it over dinner was different. It was intimate, special, reassuring to know that the memories were safe and secure inside Berra's head.

It was a delight for Guidry to listen to Berra talk about catching the old Yankees pitchers, most of all Ford. One night Berra recounted a game against the White Sox in which the first four batters reached base on four pitches—single, hit by pitch, double, and home run. On his way to the mound, manager Casey Stengel met Berra halfway and asked how Ford's stuff looked. "How the hell would I know?" Berra said. "I haven't caught one yet."

Guidry laughed and thought, *Some things in baseball never do change.* Berra's story reminded him of the time he surrendered three solid hits to the first three batters in the first inning. When he turned around, he found Thurman Munson right in his face. "Do you want me to stop telling 'em what's coming?" Munson asked. Like Berra with Vic Raschi, Munson must have known that Guidry pitched better when riled. He struck out the next three hitters.

The more he and Berra went out, the more fascinated Guidry became with the history of all things Yogi and Yankees, and that was why he seldom talked about himself. "I don't see the logic in that, because my stuff is incomparable to his," he said. "That's just how I feel." Besides, Guidry figured, what could he possibly tell Berra about his own career that Berra hadn't already seen for himself?

On top of that, the more questions he asked, the brighter the twinkle in Berra's eyes got. "As much as we talked about baseball, he really perked up when he talked about his grandchildren — so I would ask him if he had a favorite," Guidry said.

"Nah, they're all good kids," Berra would say.

"And then he liked talking about being a kid himself in St. Louis, playing make-believe games, coming from a big Italian family, talking about himself in another time, which maybe he doesn't get to do too much," Guidry said. "You know how that gets — someone gets a little older, and everyone is too busy to listen."

That was the beauty of spring training for Guidry, who preferred a slower pace — his life in Louisiana versus the rat race of New York. His time in Tampa felt unhurried: sunny days around the Yankees' complex, maybe a couple of hours on the golf course, a good meal out with a great man.

For Berra, the feeling was mutual. What could be better than a shot of Ketel One to take the edge off things, a look at the menu, and then dinner with the most attentive battery mate he could possibly have for a metaphorical game of pitch and catch?

Like Berra, Guidry is not a boastful man, but he is a proud man, well versed in heritage and history. His family roots can be traced to French settlers in Nova Scotia known as Acadians, who were persecuted by the British. Refusing to renounce their Catholicism, the Acadians staged years-long protests that eventually were met with brutal repression. In the mid-eighteenth century, they were violently driven from the island.

Those who survived the grueling move south found refuge deep in the heart of Louisiana. Out of swampland, the Acadians — shortened to "Cajuns" — built a spirited homeland with their unique culture and cuisine. They became known for their earthiness and commitment to family and were easily identified by their French traditions and heavily accented speech.

Hence, Guidry could relate to Berra when he spoke of how his immigrant parents, Pietro and Paulina, had settled in the tight-knit St. Louis neighborhood of narrow row houses called the Hill — or Dago Hill, by the ignorant and intolerant. He instantly admired the long-deceased Pietro Berra, who had left the poor tenant farms of northern Italy for the promise of America and a grueling but steady factory job producing bricks and other clay products.

Guidry's father, Roland, was also a laborer, on freight trains making their way across the bayous. Later he became a conductor on the Amtrak line from Lafayette to Houston. As a boy, Guidry loved trains, and now he was riveted by Berra's rhapsodizing about his days riding the rails early in his career with the Yankees. Those teams, he insisted, were all the closer for the endless hours they spent playing cards and sharing meals and just about everything else that fraternal young men have in common.

"We were like a family, real close-knit, always pulling for each other, always looking out for one another — on and off the field," Berra said. "Everybody got along; everybody fit in."

Guidry also believed in the bonding power of trains, having experienced it with his father. Even after he had achieved full-blown stardom with the Yankees, he would make the run with Roland — who long answered to the nickname "Rags" — during the off-season as a way of making up for lost time. After months in the air, he enjoyed the relaxed simplicity, the earthbound views. He was proud of his father's work, as was Berra, who learned about discipline and punctuality in the perfunctory act of providing a cold beer for Pietro when he got home from work.

The youngest of four Berra boys, Lawrence had to drop whatever he was doing — including the bat if he was playing ball in the neighborhood—when he heard the factory whistle at 4:30 P.M. The beer glass had to be on the kitchen table before his father stepped into the house. There was no excuse for being late.

Pietro Berra was Old World all the way, demanding that his sons learn a trade, find a job, and leave children's games like baseball behind. Yogi's brothers all played ball recreationally, and one in particular—Tony, known as "Lefty"—was good enough to earn an invitation to try out with the Cleveland Indians, if only his father had allowed it.

There was a time in Guidry's young life when it looked as if he, too, would be forbidden to play baseball. As a boy, his mother's brother had been hospitalized for a lengthy period with a baseball injury. Worse, the death of another local boy after being hit with a ball in the heart had traumatized Grace Guidry. She looked at her only child—small for his age and frail—and told him that he should be content with watching the Yankees on television alongside her.

The story Guidry likes to tell is that he remained on the sidelines until the day he walked past a ball field and picked up a ball that had rocketed past the outfielders. Without so much as a stride—as he recalled it—his throw reached home plate on the fly. One of the coaches soon begged Roland to let his boy play. After a week or two of secret practices, father and son appealed to Grace, who finally agreed but would leave the field and sit in the car when skinny little Ronnie came in from the outfield to pitch.

In Berra's case, he was forever indebted to his older brothers, who not only made a left-handed hitter out of a natural righty but relentlessly lobbied their father to allow him to pursue the opportunity denied them. "If it wasn't for my brothers, I'd probably have worked in a shoe factory or something," Yogi told Guidry, adding that his father—much like Grace Guidry—eventually came around and realized that baseball was not just a game in America; it was a passion and a pastime. When Berra asked his father to imagine how much money the family might have made if all four brothers had played ball, Pietro said, "Blame your mother."

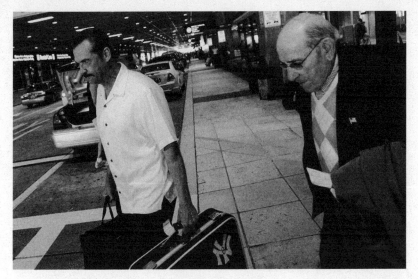

Yogi Berra could always count on Ron Guidry to be on time and to carry his bags.

(Edward Linsmier / *New York Times*)

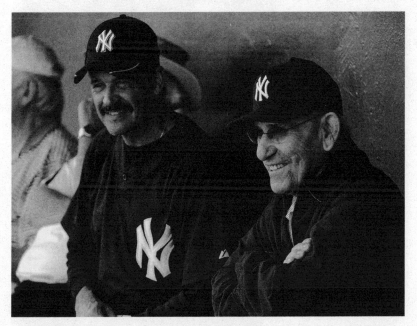

Close friends, side by side in the Yankees' dugout, taking in a spring training game.

(Barton Silverman / *New York Times*)

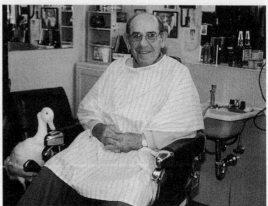

Yogi starring in his celebrated "affliction" (actually Aflac) commercial.

(Courtesy of the Yogi Berra Museum & Learning Center)

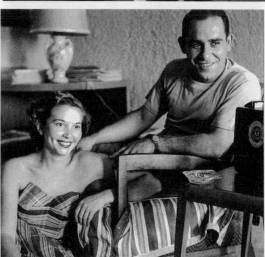

Yogi and Carmen Berra, the picture of 1950s American suburban bliss.

(Courtesy of the Yogi Berra Museum & Learning Center)

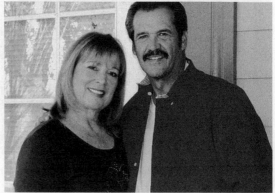

Ron and Bonnie Guidry, hometown sweethearts from Cajun country in Louisiana.

(Danielle Guidry)

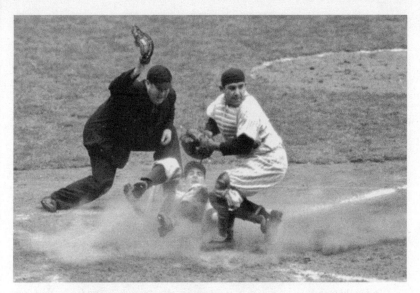

After registering an out at the plate, the catlike Berra wheels, looking for another.

(Courtesy of the Yogi Berra Museum & Learning Center)

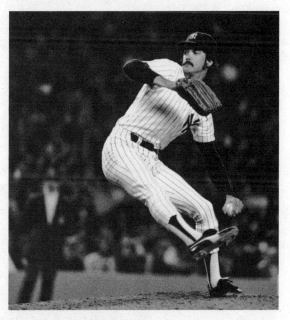

Ron Guidry as "Louisiana Lightning," pitching for the Yankees.

(Associated Press)

Berra shares a laugh with George Steinbrenner on the night the Boss begged his forgiveness at Berra's museum in New Jersey.

(Arthur Krasinsky)

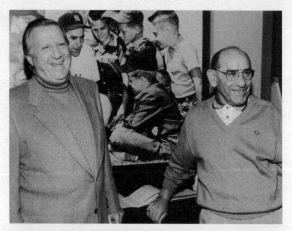

Catcher Joe Girardi asked for a blessing on his glove on Yogi Berra Day. David Cone promptly threw a perfect game as Berra and Don Larsen looked on.

(Courtesy of the Yogi Berra Museum & Learning Center)

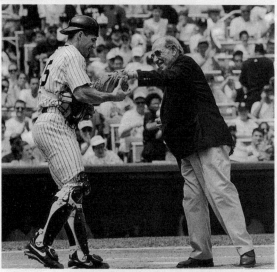

The custom-made "Driving Mr. Yogi" cap that Guidry—Berra's self-described valet—wore with pride.

(Edward Linsmier / New York Times)

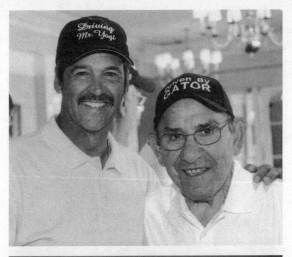

Berra had a cap of his own, inscribed "Driven by Gator."

(Courtesy of the Yogi Berra Museum & Learning Center)

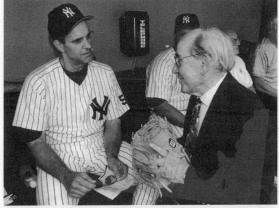

Joe Torre begged Berra to hand out 1996 championship rings to the Yankees and fussed over him when he finally returned to the team in 2000.

(Courtesy of the Yogi Berra Museum & Learning Center)

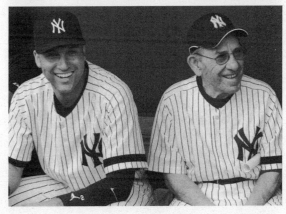

Berra was one of the few people with enough clout to penetrate Derek Jeter's defenses and form an affectionate, playful relationship with the shortstop.

(John Munson / *Star Ledger* / Corbis)

In his first spring training back with the Yankees, Berra wanted to "learn" Jorge Posada his experience, as Bill Dickey once did for him.

(Courtesy of the Yogi Berra Museum & Learning Center)

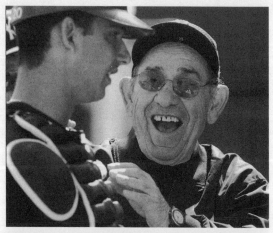

Berra helped Nick Swisher with his stroke, and Swisher gave his surrogate grandfather a hand with his uniform shirt buttons.

(New York Yankees)

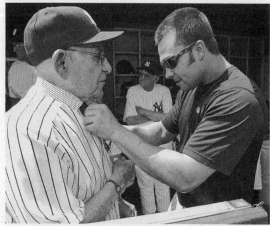

Ron Guidry found a like-minded Yankee in the great closer Mariano Rivera.

(Steve Nesius / Reuters / Corbis)

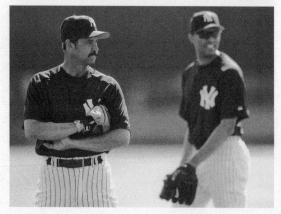

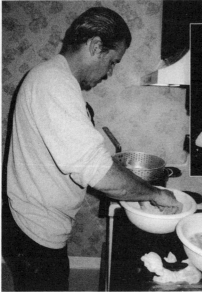

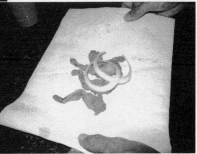

A small serving of Guidry's specialty—not enough to satisfy Berra's hearty appetite for them. (Lily Hawryluk)

When Guidry cooked his famous frog legs, Berra wanted the kitchen cleared so the master chef could focus. (Lily Hawryluk)

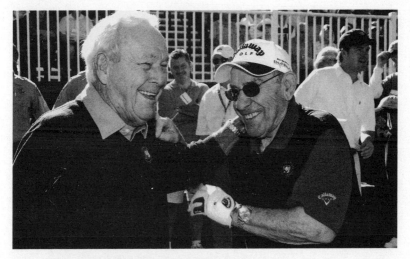

Before having to retire his clubs, Berra had golfed with the greats of the game—shown here with Arnold Palmer—and a few presidents, too.

(Bob Hope Classic Picture Library)

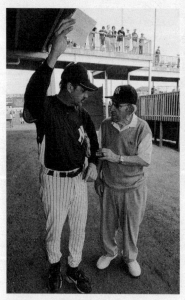

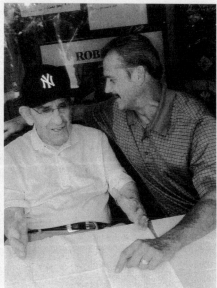

Berra and Guidry at spring training 2011, when Yogi asked for Gator's permission not to suit up anymore.

(Barton Silverman / *New York Times*)

At an autograph show in Cooperstown, New York, July 2011, Guidry made sure that Berra got his rest on an oppressively hot afternoon.

(Herbert Rein)

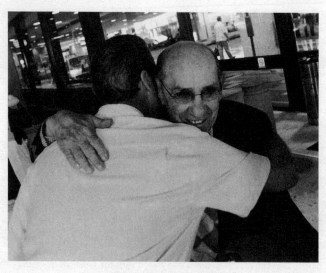

Saying goodbye, until next year.

(Edward Linsmier / *New York Times*)

SHARED VALUES • 85

Berra survived his parents' objections, but he found he had to overcome even greater challenges, in the baseball experts who doubted he was major-league material. The most famous of them was Branch Rickey. The Brooklyn Dodgers' brilliant judge of talent refused to sign the teenage Berra after a tryout at Sportsman's Park in St. Louis, saying that no kid who was all of five feet seven and not exactly built for speed would ever be more than a minor-leaguer.

Though temporarily deflated by Rickey's evaluation, Berra wound up with the same $500 signing bonus from the Yankees that his boyhood pal Joe Garagiola earned from the hometown Cardinals. But even as a minor-leaguer, Berra said, "nobody took me seriously." When he returned to the United States after serving in World War II and was assigned to a submarine base in New London, Connecticut, he was laughed at when he said he was the property of the New York Yankees. The manager of the base team told him he looked like a wrestler.

"Maybe being in a sailor suit didn't help," he admitted to Guidry. "I guess I looked worse in mine than most guys and smaller than I really was."

When Berra joined the Yankees in the spring of 1947, the reporters were the worst critics of all. Petty to the point of being cruel, they called him Quasimodo and said it was a good thing he was a catcher and would be wearing a mask.

There were mean jokes about his perceived intelligence. After he was hit in the head with a ball during practice and carried off the field on a stretcher, one wise guy wrote, "X-rays of his head showed nothing."

"I can believe that," Guidry said, shaking his head with a flash of anger in his eyes. He had experienced firsthand how mean-spirited coverage of the Yankees could be.

On another level, he was amazed by how matter-of-fact Berra could be when discussing the slings and arrows that had to be piercing for a young man starting out in the world. Yes, it was ancient history, long since survived and surmounted, but it occurred to Guidry that Berra must have had an incredibly thick skin, an innate ability to ignore the gibes and keep moving forward.

The more he heard about Berra's past, the more Guidry's chest swelled — for Berra and for himself. He, too, had dealt with a fair amount of skepticism regarding his chances of becoming a major-league pitcher. Soon after hanging up the phone with a scout named Atlee Donald, who'd informed him that he had been taken by the Yankees in the third round of the 1971 amateur draft, Grace Guidry had said, "You're joking." She had never imagined her son making a career of baseball.

No one ever poked fun at Guidry's looks, however. He was a handsome and popular high school baseball player and track star, capable of running a 9.8-second 100 and a 49-flat 440 and triple-jumping 45 feet. Guidry may have been a lightweight in the power pitcher division, but he was as fine-tuned and muscularly proportioned an athlete as anyone who ever stepped inside a baseball clubhouse.

Still, as fast as he could run and as hard as he could throw, many people — George Steinbrenner among them — just couldn't imagine Guidry as a successful starting pitcher until he was one. How, they asked, could a man under six feet with the frame of a cyclist throw in the midnineties and possibly last for up to nine innings?

Guidry and Berra both drew satisfaction from conclusively demonstrating that there was much more to the game than the perfect body type. In Guidry's mind, this only strengthened their bond.

"Guys like him and I, we get no more pleasure from anything than proving people wrong," Guidry said. "A lot of people think they know something, and they don't know crap. I don't know what makes planes fly. I don't know why rockets can go to the moon. But just because I'm small doesn't mean that I can't throw nine innings.

"When I would hear Yogi talk about himself, I remembered feeling the same thing. Our thoughts were on the same level. Nobody was going to tell us that we couldn't do the job. We knew they were wrong in thinking what they thought about us because if somebody is telling you that you're too small, well, there are a lot of things that you don't know about me. You don't know what I have experienced. You don't know what's inside of me. You don't know where I come from."

The southern terminus for Interstate 49 just happens to be Guidry's hometown of Lafayette, Louisiana. Not that he asked for that number when he joined the Yankees in 1975. Pete Sheehy, the Yankees' clubhouse man going back to the days of Ruth and Gehrig, handed him the uniform and said, "No one's ever worn it before. Take it and make it famous."

Guidry proceeded to do enough in number 49 to get it retired by the Yankees in 2003 and to earn a plaque in Yankee Stadium's Monument Park, if not in the Hall of Fame in Cooperstown. With twenty-twenty hindsight, one might consider the number coincidence a sign that Guidry was meant to be a big-league star.

To some people, it might have sounded strange when Guidry referred to Berra as his best friend, since Yogi was twenty-five years his senior. Guidry, in fact, was born only months after Larry Berra, Yogi's oldest son. Yes, they were bonded as proud, champion Yankees, but that didn't get to the heart of their relationship. Perhaps more than baseball itself, what they most shared was their personal values, lives anchored in the proverbial American dream.

In 1955, Main Street, U.S.A., was introduced to Yogi Berra, family man, during a nationally televised Edward R. Murrow *Person to Person* segment. The cameras found the man who had been derided as Quasimodo to be the picture of suburban bliss, with a beautiful wife and two sons. (Carmen Berra would carry their third child to Don Larsen's perfect game one year later and promise to name him Dale if the Dodgers' Dale Mitchell cooperated by making the last out.)

When Berra was fired as the Yankees' manager in 1964, he had offers to manage elsewhere, thanks to ninety-nine wins and reaching the seventh game of the World Series. He instead took a coaching job with the lowly New York Mets because he "didn't want to uproot

Carm and the kids, make them go to a new school in a strange place."
He stayed home in New Jersey until the Astros hired him as a coach
in 1986, long after his sons were out on their own.

The Berra boys all settled within a few miles of their parents, the
family ultimately expanding to include eleven grandchildren. Most
holidays, especially Thanksgiving, were celebrated at Carmen and
Yogi's Montclair home.

When Guidry visited each year to play in Berra's annual charity
golf tournament, usually held in early June, he couldn't help but be reminded of his own home life. The terrain and culture were different;
the pace of life was faster; and the housing lots were certainly smaller
than the property he lived on. But the family structure was not unlike
the one he and Bonnie had built a short drive into the country from
downtown Lafayette, in the neighboring township of Scott.

Off commercial Route 93, dotted with HAY FOR SALE and other
farm-related signs, the turnoff for the Guidry homestead is a narrow road, Rue Novembre. The landscape itself is flat enough so that
Guidry can point to an intersection far across his property in the direction of where his parents live, a short drive away.

When he lost grandparents on his paternal and maternal sides and
the surviving spouses were reluctant to move from their longtime
residences, Guidry had both houses lifted off their lots and relocated
so they could be closer to family. He moved Bonnie's aging parents
into a small house on his own property, and when they passed away,
his daughter Jamie and her husband moved in. They had a daughter,
Ava, the Guidrys' first grandchild, in the spring of 2011. Their other
daughter, Danielle, remains in the area. Only their son, Brandon, has
left, taking up residence in New York.

The family is not large, although there are several hundred
Guidrys listed in the area phone book. During his baseball-playing
years, fan mail would occasionally come from other Guidrys wondering if they were related to the suddenly famous Ron. Rags Guidry
joked that with each succeeding victory, people claiming to be his
son's third cousins would become second cousins, and so on.

Like Berra, Guidry married his hometown sweetheart, Bonnie Rutledge, in 1972. He was twenty-two; she was eighteen. Their first residence was an apartment behind his parents' home, which was fine with Guidry. Other than the pitcher's mound at Yankee Stadium, he never aspired to be anywhere other than Lafayette, a city of about 120,000. That was why he wasn't bitter when the Yankees cut him loose as a pitcher. Like Berra in 1964 and again in 1985, he at least got to go home, financially secure, and what was so bad about that?

"It's quiet here, and that's what I love," Guidry said, welcoming a visitor to an old barn he calls "the doghouse." It contains all the trappings — tools, tractor, pool table, finished room with a small kitchen and a large-screen TV — of the proverbial man cave.

With his lyrical Cajun accent and his fondness for keeping a spittoon nearby, Guidry has old-fashioned hardball written all over him. He has been an avid hunter almost since he could lift a gun and his paternal grandfather, Gus, took him out in the woods. He is not shy about sprinkling a story with well-timed profanity. But only when the extremely private Guidry lowers his guard — when he speaks of his relationship with Berra, for instance — does his emotional complexity reveal itself.

When the Yankees drafted him in 1971, he was studying architecture at the University of Southwestern Louisiana. When his career took off in 1978, fueled by the most dominant season a Yankees starter has ever had, Guidry might have exploited the moment and cut numerous endorsement deals. He instead rejected offers to pitch a soft drink because it wasn't the one he preferred and a tobacco product because he didn't want to encourage young people to emulate him. He also had little patience for the self-promotional banquet circuit. It took time away from his family, especially his younger brother, Travis, with whom he spent as much time as he could during the off-season.

So excited was the seventeen-year-old Guidry when his mother told him she was pregnant with Travis that he begged his parents to let him name the baby if it was a boy. He chose Travis after Travis

Williams, the star running back of the Green Bay Packers. Guidry was ecstatic to finally have a sibling and especially a brother. But the mood changed dramatically when doctors disclosed that little Travis had been deprived of oxygen for too long during the birth and would have severe mental and physical handicaps.

Given the age difference between his brother and him, Guidry practically became a third parent. On Travis's delayed terms, Ron spent hour after hour encouraging him to walk and talk, run and throw, even shoot a gun. He understood that his brother would never navigate the world as a "normal" child, but he took pride in Travis's victories, both physical and mental, bragging about his prowess with puzzles and his knack for remembering names and faces.

Guidry has an appreciation not only for the small pleasures of life but also for life itself. The birth of his first grandchild in May 2011, for instance, was a time for celebration, but not only because of the baby's birth. Ron and Bonnie could again count their blessings for Jamie's survival of a horrific car crash when she was in high school. The police officer who found her told Guidry that his first thought when he came upon the wreckage was that there could be no survivors.

These are the victories that most sustain Guidry, the trophies he values. He insists that if it wasn't for Bonnie, the evidence of his fourteen years of major-league service would be boxed and in storage, ultimately left for the children to deal with. She insists on displaying some of it behind sliding glass doors in the den.

But even these items are not conventional trophies. Propped against the trophy case is a golf bag from Berra's charity golf tournament with his trademark logo — a silhouette of him leaning on a bat. Inside the glass are team photos of the late-seventies Yankees, candid shots of Guidry with his favorite teammates, and an enlarged box score of his first major-league game against the Red Sox at Shea Stadium in 1975 — symbolic of his long struggle to get to the big leagues and stay there.

Singled out for a visitor's attention by Guidry was a Los Angeles

Dodgers cap, a souvenir of the 1981 World Series received on an off day when the Yankees and Dodgers were working out at Dodger Stadium. Guidry was minding his own business near the dugout when he heard Jeff Torborg calling to him from the Dodgers' side of the field. Torborg was striding toward home plate with none other than Sandy Koufax.

Guidry knew Torborg, a New Jersey guy who had caught for the Dodgers and Angels in the sixties and was Koufax's battery mate when he pitched a perfect game in 1965. Koufax was taller than Guidry by three inches and in his pitching days probably outweighed him by forty pounds. But he apparently had noticed similarities in their pitching styles, as had others. As they came face-to-face for the first time at home plate — Guidry on the Yankees' side, Koufax on the Dodgers' — Koufax held out his hand and said, "I marvel at the way you pitch. I watch you as much as I can."

"That's really nice of you to say," Guidry said, startled and hoping not to blush.

"I'm not in the habit of asking a Yankee for an autograph, but I was wondering if you'd be willing to exchange autographed caps," Koufax said.

Guidry grabbed the cap with the interlocking "LA" logo and surrendered his own before Koufax could change his mind. Koufax's inscription read, "To Ron: Good luck and very best wishes — Sandy Koufax."

Guidry rushed to the clubhouse to put the cap away. Thirty years later, he called it his most treasured baseball keepsake.

Berra also felt a strong connection to Koufax, despite having been an opponent, though never having faced him in a game. The closest he came was at the very end of the 1963 World Series, during his final year playing for the Yankees, when he stepped into the on-deck circle to pinch hit with two outs and two on in the ninth inning. The Yankees were down a run to Koufax and the Dodgers and trying to avoid a four-game sweep. Hector Lopez grounded out, and that was that.

Nine years later, in the class of 1972, Berra was thrilled to be inducted into the Hall of Fame with Koufax. When he and Guidry were out one night, he said that he sure wished he could have faced the great Dodger from Brooklyn in his final at bat for the Yankees, whatever the outcome would have been.

Seizing the moment for pitchers everywhere, poking Berra as he took every opportunity to do, Guidry shot him a look as if to say, *Like there would have been any doubt?*

7

Total Recall

The first thing Yogi Berra typically did after settling into his hotel room in Tampa was remember everything he had forgotten.

Mouthwash. Shaving cream. Q-tips. Packs of Dentyne to last him over the coming weeks.

"Gator, I gotta go shopping," he'd say.

Off they would go to the nearest supermarket, where Berra could also pick up cold cuts, bread, and assorted treats for those evenings when Guidry decided he needed a night off from the restaurant rotation.

So there they were one afternoon, the septuagenarian and the fiftysomething Guidry, pushing a cart up and down the aisles of the neighborhood 7-Eleven, with Guidry thinking Berra had everything he needed.

"Ready to check out?" he said.

"No, let's go this way," Berra said, steering the cart into another aisle, slowing to look at the items on the shelves but not taking anything off.

When he turned down another aisle, Guidry realized what Berra was up to. "You dirty old man," he said, nodding at the attractive young woman in the short sundress whom Berra was following around the store.

Berra flashed a sheepish smile that said, *OK, you got me. Guilty as charged. Sue me for not having forgotten that I was young once.*

Guidry was finding out that there was little Berra had forgotten, especially when the subject was baseball.

More than most, Don Zimmer knew how to get Berra's goat when walking down memory lane, even over a pleasant dinner out. "Watch this," he said to Guidry a few months after the Yankees had beaten the Mets in the 2000 World Series.

The buzz of New York's first "subway series" in forty-four years was still in the air, at least in that part of Tampa where proud Yankees roamed. Zimmer only qualified as a half-breed, having played for the Brooklyn and Los Angeles Dodgers and managed the Red Sox — albeit at a time, circa 1978, few people in Boston cared to remember. He'd signed on as Joe Torre's bench coach in 1996 and served as interim Yankees manager when Torre underwent treatment for prostate cancer during the 1999 season.

A character in his own right — with a nickname, "Popeye," befitting a fair facial resemblance — Zimmer lacked a notable playing resumé. Just the same, he was a beloved lifer, with the touch, tenure, and temerity to tweak Berra as often as he could.

"Yog," he said, "I don't see why you got that big picture in your museum of you and Jackie that you're always hollerin' about. You know damn well he was safe."

Berra didn't go all apoplectic on Zimmer the way he freaked out on Bill Summers — the umpire who believed he saw Jackie Robinson slide under Berra's tag while stealing home in the eighth inning of game one of the 1955 World Series. Mask in hand, Berra was right in Summers's chest and chased him several feet behind the plate to argue his case.

"How come you didn't get tossed?" Guidry asked.

"He probably knew I was right," Berra said.

When it came to the Robinson call, Berra wore his certitude like a badge of honor, even signing a photo of the play that was destined for Barack Obama with the inscription, "Dear Mr. President: He was out." He would argue that Frank Kellert, the Dodgers hitter who was at the plate at the time, had admitted to reporters that he had had the best view of the play and that Summers had gotten it wrong. Berra figured the admission at least justified the most visible outburst of his career.

Forty-five years later, Berra's resistance to any opposing view of the call was still as predictable as a pinstripe. Determined to make sure his new pal Guidry knew the score, Berra grumped at Zimmer, but Zimmer was just getting started on the subject of that series. A second-year infielder for the Dodgers at the time, he had slugged a robust 15 home runs in 280 at bats that season and had started the game because of his hitting.

Fast-forward to game seven, the Dodgers clinging to a 2–0 lead in the sixth inning behind left-hander Johnny Podres. Walter Alston, the Brooklyn manager, decided to make a defensive change in left field. Replacing Jim Gilliam with Sandy Amoros, he then moved Gilliam to second base, pulling Zimmer to keep Gilliam, one of his better players, in the game.

Billy Martin walked to lead off the inning, and Gil McDougald beat out a bunt. Then came the lefty Berra, who chased a pitch that was tailing away — no surprise for a man whose strike zone was however far he could extend the meat of the bat — and drove it down the left-field line. The ball had two-run double written all over it until Amoros, who had outstanding speed, seemingly appeared out of nowhere to make one of the great World Series catches of all time. He was able to make the grab in the corner, a few feet from the wall, only because he was left-handed and had his glove hand in perfect position.

The relay from Pee Wee Reese to Gil Hodges at first base doubled off McDougald. The Yankees mustered only one more hit after that, falling to their Brooklyn rivals for the only time in seven World Series the two teams played between 1941 and 1956. Zimmer never let Berra forget his role in bringing about Brooklyn's finest hour.

"If not for me, you'd have been a hero," he told Berra.

Berra had an effective comeback. "We got even the next year," he said, referring to the 1956 World Series, which featured Don Larsen's perfect game and two generally overlooked home runs by Berra to lead the Yankees to a 9–0 victory in another game seven.

The way Berra and Zimmer carried on reminded Guidry of the old comedy team Abbott and Costello. "I ate that up, couldn't get enough," he said.

In Guidry's view, the best stories came from the days when New York could almost count on a subway series — seven times in a ten-year period that began in Berra's first full season, 1947 — six against Brooklyn and one against the New York Giants. Considering New York's love affair with baseball, he could only imagine how intense that must have been.

"No days off, but what I liked is that we didn't have to travel — fifteen or twenty minutes, and we were there," Berra told him, referring to the team's bus ride to Ebbets Field — the slight time exaggeration beyond the point. (Even by subway, it took longer to travel from Yankee Stadium to Brooklyn.) "Everyone thinks we hated the Dodgers. We didn't. We wanted to beat them, but we got along fine. We barnstormed in the off-season, did appearances together. We were friends off the field."

To prove his point, Berra described a photo on display in his museum. He is wearing street clothes, congratulating Podres in the Dodgers' clubhouse after game seven. He especially wanted Guidry to know how much he admired Jackie Robinson, who in turn used to say that Berra was the Dodgers' most feared Yankee. Berra also forged a friendship with Dodgers catcher Roy Campanella, visiting him during the off-season at his liquor store in Harlem.

Hearing Berra and Zimmer reminisce and being something of a traditionalist himself, Guidry was left with a growing appreciation for when World Series games were played in the sunshine in about two hours' time, when the front pages of ten New York newspapers screamed the latest results and radio was still the dominant electronic medium, leaving so much to the imagination. The city came to a virtual standstill, Berra told him. "That's all everybody talked about," he said.

By October 2000, the now rare occurrence of a subway series had the New York media bathing in nostalgia, even as swaths of a city with large minority and immigrant populations wondered what the fuss was all about. Many could not identify with Willie (Mays), Mickey (Mantle), and the Duke (Snider). They knew nothing of the long-vanished Ebbets Field and Polo Grounds. But for those working the angle of postwar New York, Berra was the must-get interview. Reporters and television crews flocked to his museum to ask about Larsen, Robinson, and the rest.

Berra was psyched, nagging Dave Kaplan, often his driving companion, to leave at 1:00 P.M. for a game scheduled to begin a few minutes after 7:00. "Let's go now — it's a good time," he'd say, checking his watch. "We'll beat the traffic."

Berra would arrive so early that he would pass through a near-empty clubhouse and head straight for Joe Torre's office to turn on the lights before the manager had even stepped into the building. When his clubhouse schmoozing was done, he would head up to George Steinbrenner's box to watch the game, though Berra inevitably preferred being off in a corner by himself — muttering under his breath when the Yankees failed to deliver a runner in scoring position — to rubbing elbows with the assortment of invited glitterati.

He would typically slip out by the fifth or sixth inning, not because he was tired or bored but to beat the traffic and make it home in about twenty-five minutes, so that he could catch the last few innings in the quiet of his den, just as he had done for fourteen years. There, safely out of earshot of those who wouldn't understand that he was just an old-school lifer and hopeless Yankees fan venting his frustration over what he was watching, he could complain to his heart's content and swear that "if I was playing now I'd hit .400." If Carmen or one of their sons was nearby, they'd nod a couple of times and pay him no mind.

The 2000 World Series itself was nothing remarkable, with the Yankees winning in five games for their third straight title and fourth in five years. Derek Jeter was the MVP. Perhaps the sweetest moment of the series was with two outs in the fifth inning of game four, when a diminished David Cone threw his last pitch as a Yankee after being summoned by Torre to face Mets slugger Mike Piazza.

It had been only a year and change since his perfect game on Yogi Berra Day, but Cone was no longer in the rotation. He would forever be indebted to Torre for calling on him at all to replace the southpaw Denny Neagle, who was none too pleased to be yanked when he was one out away from a World Series victory.

At thirty-seven, Cone was pitching mostly on fumes. The best he could muster against Piazza was a mideighties fastball. But the pitch had just enough tail to get inside Piazza's big swing and cause him to pop up. Cone walked triumphantly off the mound and later would call the cameo "one of the great highlights of my career, without a doubt."

Having starred for the Mets in the eighties and the Yankees in the nineties, Cone had a better understanding than most players of what it meant to play in a subway series. "I was in the bullpen kind of like a kid looking through the glass at Shea wondering if I was going to get to play, almost wallowing in self-pity," he said. "You know, I had always dreamed about that, a subway series. Even though we played each other during the regular season, a World Series was different."

He knew how much so because he was one of the Yankees who had made it his business the previous spring and during the season to have a running dialogue with the man who owned ten World Series rings. Berra wore only the one he earned in 1953 — New York 4, Brooklyn 2 — because it represented a record fifth straight championship.

One day Cone asked him, "Didn't you guys ever get tired of beating the Dodgers?"

"Hell, no," Berra said, repeating himself for emphasis and looking surprised that Cone would even ask such a thing.

On the morning of September 11, 2001, Berra was on his way home after a workout on the treadmill and light weights at the gym. When he turned on the radio, he heard devastating news: planes had flown into the Twin Towers in New York. The Pentagon had also been hit. The nation was under attack.

From the crest of a hill on Bloomfield Avenue at the Montclair-Verona border, through the windshield of his red Jaguar, Berra now knew why smoke was darkening the sky over lower Manhattan, about fifteen miles to the east.

"How could these people do this to such innocent people?" he asked Carmen when he arrived home and watched in horror as the towers fell.

She didn't have an answer. No one did. The horror of 9/11 hit home for Berra, who had golfed with one of the World Trade Center victims at a local club. He had family connections to a few others who were lost. He openly wept at a funeral when he saw the young children there, senselessly shorn of a parent. He wished he could do something; he wanted to help. When a call came a few weeks later from the office of the mayor, Rudy Giuliani, he got his chance.

In an effort to restore the city's image and reignite the tourism industry, Giuliani reached out to several New York icons — Robert De Niro, Woody Allen, Billy Crystal, and his all-time favorite baseball player — to appear in a series of public-service commercials. The spots played on incongruity, with Berra cast as the conductor of the New York Philharmonic, all gussied up and gesticulating wildly before turning to the camera to ask, "Who in the heck is this guy Phil Harmonic?"

In the weeks after the attack, Berra was among the many athletes and celebrities who quietly accommodated numerous requests for photos, autographs, and even phone messages to widows and children. He took to wearing an American flag on the lapel of his sports jacket. When old baseball friends from around the country — Guidry included — checked in to say they were feeling New York's pain, Berra wound up consoling *them,* sharing the sense of togetherness that had spread throughout the region. The Yankees, he assured them, were helping. They were going to play, and they were going to win.

In a matter of weeks, the baseball playoffs again came to the city, but with an altered subtext of how America identified with the Yankees. This time they were not the payroll-bloated bullies. They were victims, or representatives of victims, wearing caps that honored fallen firemen and police officers.

But when they dropped the first two games of the American League Division Series to the Oakland A's at Yankee Stadium, it looked as if the much-needed diversion of postseason baseball would be short-lived. Heading out west for game three, Torre reached back for a little spiritual help from the man he perceived as a good-luck charm. He asked Berra for a different cap — one with his trademark saying, IT AIN'T OVER 'TIL IT'S OVER — that was marketed and sold by his sons.

Torre had the "NYPD" logo stitched into the side of the cap and wore it to every batting practice and pregame press conference for the remainder of October — and into November. The Yankees honored the prophet Berra and the fighting spirit of the city with a stirring comeback against the A's.

Mike Mussina had the assignment of starting game three and keeping the Yankees alive. This was Mussina's first season with the club; he wore number 35 and would never forget his introduction to Berra after he was helped into his new jersey at the press conference to formally announce his signing.

"You got my number," Berra told Mussina.

Mussina, a Stanford man and *New York Times* crossword puzzle connoisseur, knew his famous baseball numbers. But Yogi Berra — 35? He was dumbfounded.

"I wore thirty-five my rookie year, 1947," Berra told him.

This was one piece of trivia that Mussina didn't know.

"Wow, really?" he said, already feeling better about his decision to become a Yankee.

In Oakland, Mussina was locked in a pitchers' duel with Barry Zito, leading 1–0 in the bottom of the seventh inning. With two outs and Jeremy Giambi on first base, Terrence Long hit a drive into the right-field corner. It appeared that Giambi, not a fast runner, would score easily when the right fielder, Shane Spencer, missed the cutoff man with his throw. But Derek Jeter, sprinting across the diamond in the vicinity of the first-base line, suddenly had the ball cradled in his midsection and somehow shoveled it to catcher Jorge Posada, who tagged a stunned Giambi as he tried to jump over the tag instead of sliding around it.

Jeter's intervention was instantly hailed as one of the great improvisational plays in postseason history, but he refused credit for his intuitive positioning. He said the idea of stationing the shortstop near the first-base line on balls hit to deep right field was Don Zimmer's. Berra was right: Yankees young and old were pitching in.

Jeter's play preserved the victory and was the pivotal moment of the best-of-five series. The Yankees proceeded to take out the Seattle Mariners — winners of 116 games during the regular season — in the best-of-seven championship series in five games.

But it was their ninth-inning rallies against the Arizona Diamondbacks — astonishing because they occurred on consecutive World Series nights — that would do more to create a joyous soundtrack in a heartbroken city than anything else. Their resolve was pitch-perfect in the aftermath of 9/11, and so riveting were games four and five that even Berra didn't dare leave Yankee Stadium early.

"I don't remember the stadium ever being so loud — the building was shaking," he said when Guidry — who of course was watching in Louisiana — asked the following spring what those nights were like.

For the sake of the city's psyche, if not rabid Yankees fans, it was almost as if the series ended when Alfonso Soriano singled in Chuck Knoblauch in the twelfth inning of game five. When play shifted back to Arizona, the Yankees were blown out in game six and lost game seven excruciatingly, with Mariano Rivera on the mound, three outs away from a fourth straight World Series victory.

That it happened far away in the middle of a desert, and with the gaping wound in lower Manhattan still smoking, made it easy for Berra to put the loss in perspective. As far as he was concerned, the Yankees had risen to the occasion, done what they had needed to do.

In the years to follow, it would become a pattern—a newsreel of breathtaking postseason games but no World Series victory for a franchise that insisted that no season could be considered a success without a championship. But there was always their storied past to draw on, always someone from another decade to bring back, to keep the fans feeling nostalgic and to send a subliminal message to the new, ringless Yankees: the same ceremonial salute will be waiting for you someday if you give us the championships we crave.

Ron Guidry's day in the Yankee Stadium sun occurred on August 23, 2003. When he realized that the ceremony was not just to retire his number but also to grant him permanent residency in Monument Park, the most hallowed of Yankee Stadium neighborhoods, with his good friend Yogi and all the other franchise greats, he began to cry.

Bonnie Guidry always believed the Yankees would retire her husband's number, if only because they had never let anyone else wear it after he retired. But when the call came with the news that the organization wanted to do more, she decided to let it be a surprise. She swore her three children to secrecy, and somehow they managed to keep quiet.

Guidry walked into the stadium that day thinking the ceremony would be a routine acknowledgment that he had done with number 49 what Pete Sheehy had told him to do: "Make it famous."

Former teammates were on hand to present him with a variety of gifts—including a tractor that rolled down the warning track in right field. Reggie Jackson handed him the framed 49 jersey. And then a drape with the interlocking "NY" logo fell away, and Guidry realized that the bronze plaque that had been hidden behind it was for him. His face turned pale. He bowed his head and wiped away tears.

"Really, I would have been happy if they had just given me my jersey and said nobody's wearing it no more," he said. "But when I saw the plaque, it was like, Jesus Christ. It never dawned on me, the ultimate compliment. That's when it really hit me that I was going to be out there with Yogi and everyone."

After the legends Berra, Ford, Rizzuto, and Mattingly gathered around him for a photo, Guidry told reporters that he never believed he had done enough "to deserve what happened to me today." Most scoffed at the thought, knowing that his 154–67 record between 1977 and 1985 reflected a lengthy period of dominance that compared, at least on a percentage basis, to the six years of Sandy Koufax's career in which he went 129–47, which eventually won him election to the Hall of Fame.

"Heck, Gator won twenty-five games one year and helped us win two championships," Berra said. "He was pretty darn good, pitched real good in the postseason, too. He was as good a fielder as any pitcher I ever saw."

Guidry, Berra pointed out, was such a crowd pleaser that he started the trend of two-strike clapping at the stadium in anticipation of the strikeout. In other words, in Berra's opinion, he didn't have to apologize for his ticket to Monument Park.

The Hall of Fame was another matter, though. As a member of the Veterans Committee, Berra had helped his good friend Phil Rizzuto get elected in 1994. The committee voted on players whose eligibility for the normal nominating process — in which sportswriters and other media members presided over elections — had long since expired. Berra was so elated when the veterans voted Rizzuto in, he called the Scooter at home and told him, simply: "You're in." He also believed that Rizzuto deserved the honor. But as a general rule, he didn't enjoy commenting on players' credentials, not wanting to sound critical of anyone — even sportswriters, who were often convenient targets for a verbal thrashing. (He happened to have one in the family — his granddaughter Lindsay, who had begun reporting for *ESPN The Magazine* in 1999.)

So on the subject of whether Guidry deserved to make the Hall of Fame someday, Berra was content to say that he would have had a better chance if he had reached the majors sooner than he did. "He would've had a lot more wins," he reasoned. "That's a lot of what the writers decide on."

Guidry never gave much thought to what might have been, only what was, and in 2003 that was more than good enough for him. Eight years later, in the summer of 2011, his voice still choked with emotion as he recalled how Berra had patted him gently on the shoulder that day, telling him how much he deserved the honor but advising him to keep his speech short, because "no one wants to hear you go on and on."

In the ensuing years, the gesture would mean even more as their relationship continued to grow. Guidry loved the idea of them being together in Monument Park forever. "He's out there. I'm out there," Guidry said. "It just can't get any better than that."

More than anyone in New York, Berra knew that even when things looked bleakest for the Yankees against the Red Sox, it just meant the inevitable suffering of New England was going to be worse. In fact, he was willing to guarantee it.

"Relax," he told Bernie Williams in 1999 before another October showdown between the American League powers that would rile up the northeastern seaboard. "We've played these guys for eighty years. They can't beat us."

But on October 16, 2003, the Sox were so close to defeating the Yankees in game seven of the American League Championship Series, they could practically feel the victory champagne stinging their eyes. With a 5–2 lead after seven and a half innings and their best pitcher, Pedro Martinez, on the mound, the Boston grounds crew was feeling mighty slick about audaciously painting the World Series logo on the Fenway Park grass hours before the Sox chased their former ace Roger Clemens from the mound.

They should have known better. Soon Sox manager Grady Little — cast as a twenty-first-century Zimmer — was making a fateful trip to the mound and allowing a tiring Martinez to remain in the game. A barrage of hits later, the game was tied. Three innings after that, Aaron Boone — a Yankee since late July — hit a pennant-winning home run into the left-field seats.

It was another remarkable blow by an unremarkable Yankee. Like Bucky Dent in 1978, Boone would be forever tagged with a middle name that rhymed with ducking. Bucky Bleeping Dent, meet Aaron Bleeping Boone.

Imagine that, Berra told Guidry when he returned to spring training the following spring, sitting around the coaches' room across the hall from the clubhouse one February morning. He let everyone know that he had strolled over to Boone a few days before the home run to tell him how much he had liked his grandfather, Ray, a rival with the Cleveland Indians.

Guidry couldn't let the opportunity to roll his eyes in mock exasperation pass. "Goddamn, Yogi, you're taking credit for that, too?" he asked.

The truth was that Guidry was just superstitious enough to believe that Berra's magic could be contagious — though only to a point. Just as they had in 2001, the Yankees lost the World Series in 2003 to a team that hadn't even existed when Guidry was playing, much less Berra. Worse, the Florida Marlins had a payroll less than half that of New York. Yet they came into Yankee Stadium and wrapped up the series in six games behind the young right-handed power pitcher Josh Beckett.

Still, there wasn't quite the pall over the spring training complex in 2004 that one would have expected for a team that had failed in its annual mission to win it all. One reason was that George Stein-brenner's health was declining and he was no longer a looming, impe-rious presence. Another was that the Yankees had beaten the Red Sox again — torn their hearts out, really — and that was no inconsequen-tial achievement, given that the animosity between the teams seemed more intense than ever.

Even Guidry, who had watched the ALCS from home in Louisiana, had to admit that he had never seen anything quite like the bench-clearing fiasco in game three that had resulted in the seventy-two-year-old Zimmer charging Martinez and being flung to the ground like an old beanbag. It was mortifying, and Zimmer was fortunate to have escaped serious injury.

But if he was going to be honest about it, Guidry couldn't imagine the rivalry any other way. After all, he had joined the Yankees when it was all fear, loathing, and fisticuffs. In his experience, just beating the Red Sox wasn't enough. Crushing them was almost a sport in itself, and if it could be accomplished inside a deflated Fenway Park, all the better.

In the months after Boone's home run — and his unceremonious departure from the Yankees following an off-season injury sustained while playing basketball — tormenting the Red Sox was understand-ably a popular topic around the spring training complex. For guest instructors like Guidry and Goose Gossage, it was the perfect op-portunity to fill the coaches' room with tales of their own proudest hours — beginning with early September 1978, when they went into Boston four games behind the Sox after being down fourteen and swept them four straight by the aggregate score of 42–9.

Berra remembered the so-called Fenway Massacre well, having had a great view of it from the dugout. But he enjoyed hearing Guidry recount the old war stories again with such devilish pride. He knew from his own playing experiences that ballplayers never tire of reliv-ing them.

"The fans are booing, they're screaming, they're calling us all kinds of names. We're getting pelted with batteries and darts and ball bearings," Guidry said. "It's OK, no big deal: wear a helmet, wear a long-sleeved shirt, wear a jacket. We're going to beat the dog shit out of them anyway."

In the third game of that series, Guidry pitched a two-hit shutout for his twenty-first victory, toying with what he called "the toughest lineup I've ever faced." Three weeks later, pitching on short rest against the Sox in the one-game playoff for the pennant, he took a 4–2 lead into the seventh inning. He got the first out, gave up an opposite-field single to George Scott, and looked up to see his manager, Bob Lemon, on his way to the mound.

Guidry had never been an outspoken man who would go out of his way to seek the limelight. Many players and reporters felt as though they didn't know him at all. But inside the circle of trust, he could be the life of the party, a delightful storyteller, with his charming Cajun accent for spice and a demonstrative style that included sound effects for moments such as bat meeting ball.

In the coaches' room that spring, Guidry reminded everyone of how pissed he was when Lemon told him that he was bringing Gossage in with eight outs to go. Guidry thought he deserved the chance to get through the seventh inning. If it had been Billy Martin managing, Guidry might have said, "You need to get your ass off my mound so I can pitch."

Martin, who wouldn't back down from a tornado, had trusted Guidry to be honest about his arm. But Martin had been forced to resign in late July after his infamous comment, "One's a born liar, the other's convicted," referring first to Reggie Jackson and then to George Steinbrenner (for pleading guilty in 1974 to making illegal contributions to Richard Nixon's reelection campaign).

Lemon was not above deferring to Guidry either, but not that day with so much at stake. He took the ball while Guidry cussed a blue streak.

"I saved the damn game, didn't I?" Gossage interjected, reminding Guidry how he'd gotten Carl Yastrzemski to pop up for the last out — a showdown he had actually imagined and relished while falling asleep the night before.

"Yeah, we won the game, but you nearly gave everyone a stroke," Guidry said. "Two runs in the next inning and guys on base in the ninth."

Guidry turned to Berra. "Right, Yogi?"

Berra smiled and shot him a "whatever you say, Gator" nod. He enjoyed the raucous banter; it was like watching his sons arm-wrestle for his attention.

The truth was that Berra, thrilled as he was when the Yankees pulled out the 2003 ALCS, was saddened by what he had seen in Boston in game three. The sight of Zimmer tumbling onto the grass was especially troubling. No matter how intense, the game should never have come to that.

"You can't get caught up in it like the fans do," he said. "The fans make it life-and-death. We liked playing in that atmosphere. It was fun. But we didn't hate them; they were good guys — [Bobby] Doerr, [Johnny] Pesky, [Ted] Williams."

In fact, when Doerr got his two thousandth hit in a game against the Yankees in 1951 — the third active player at the time to reach that milestone — Berra called time-out to get the ball. He gave it to Doerr, who retired prematurely two months later with a bad back and treasured that ball into his nineties.

Above all, and from their earliest dinners out, Guidry knew better than anyone how much Berra respected Williams — how in their post-playing days they became close, how Berra sent his oldest son to Williams's baseball camp in New Hampshire, how a wheelchair-bound Williams came to Berra's museum to help launch it. Berra was almost in awe of Williams, who won the Triple Crown in Berra's rookie season and, taking one look at his squat body behind the plate, cracked, "Who in hell are the Yankees trying to fool with this guy?"

As a former pitcher from a later generation, Guidry was less interested in Williams's wisecracks than he was in hearing about how the Yankees tried to get Williams out.

Guidry: "What'd you throw him?"

Berra: "You just threw some pitches away and let him hit a lousy single. He wasn't a fast runner, so even if he hits the ball the other way — especially in Fenway, it's off the wall — you can hold him to a single."

Guidry: "What else?"

Berra: "You really focused on getting everybody in front of him out so he doesn't drive in any runs."

Guidry: "That's it?"

Berra: "No matter what, he's gonna hit. You try to talk to him and get him off his game."

Guidry: "What did you say?"

Berra: "'Done any fishing lately? Been to any good restaurants?'"

Guidry: "What would he say?"

Berra: "'Shut up, you little Dago, I'm trying to hit.'"

Guidry: "Did you ever get him to respond?"

Berra: "Oh, yeah. One time we threw him a called strike, and he kept telling me the pitch was an inch outside."

Guidry: "What did you say?"

Berra: "'If I had those good pitches to swing at, I'd be a rich guy like you.'"

Guidry: "Who was better, Williams or DiMaggio?"

Berra: "Oh, Joe D."

Guidry: "Why was that?"

Berra: "Williams was the best hitter I ever saw. Joe was the best player and, you know . . ."

Guidry: "What?"

Berra: "Well, we always won."

If Guidry and Gossage relished 1978 and Jeter and Rivera savored 2003, Berra had 1949. Long before Bucky Dent and Aaron Boone, the

Red Sox managed to lose the race that season to a Yankees team that was plagued by injuries and forced to play without an aging DiMaggio for a spell in September due to a bout with pneumonia.

The Red Sox, who the previous season had lost the pennant to Cleveland in a one-game playoff, appeared to be on a mission. Mel Parnell, their ace, had a 25-win season. Ellis Kinder won 23. Williams drove in 159 runs, a monster sum that was equaled by a teammate, infielder Vern Stephens.

Having taken sole possession of first place from the Yankees just days before by rallying from a 6–3 deficit, the Red Sox pulled into New York on October 1 for the season-ending two-game series, needing one win to clinch. DiMaggio returned to the lineup on a day the Yankees celebrated his career with one of their gift-laden ceremonies, after which DiMaggio thanked everyone, including "the good Lord for making me a Yankee." His most famous quotation gave the young Berra goose bumps.

But the Red Sox proceeded to knock Allie Reynolds out in the third inning, grabbing the same 4–0 lead behind Parnell that Martinez would be given in 2003. Parnell's didn't last even as long as Martinez's. Playing with a sore hand, Berra knocked in a run with a double as the Yankees tied the game in the fifth. They won it in the eighth on the sixth home run of the season by Johnny Lindell, a journeyman outfielder and onetime pitcher who hit .242 that year.

Johnny Bleeping Lindell!

With the rivals deadlocked on the final day of the season, the Yankees were facing Kinder. They managed to carry a 1–0 lead into the eighth inning behind Vic Raschi. That inning, they exploded for four runs and held on to win 5–3, though not before DiMaggio bizarrely removed himself from the game after failing to catch a long drive by Doerr that went for a triple. The series attracted almost 140,000 fans to Yankee Stadium. The year before Guidry was born, Casey Stengel won his first pennant as Yankees manager, and Berra's sense of manifest destiny was shaped.

"All they had to do was win one of two games," he told Guidry, breaking down Boston's misery to simple math. "They didn't."

Or couldn't. And the most unbelievable part of it all was that Williams could muster just one hit in the series and failed to drive in a single run. All in the spirit of good, clean competition, Berra had much more to talk about when Teddy Ballgame came to the plate in 1950.

When it finally happened, it felt like a dream, almost surreal, like watching an episode of *The Twilight Zone*. One minute the Yankees were almost mocking the Red Sox in the 2004 American League Championship Series, blowing them out three games to none. The next minute the Red Sox were running away with game seven, and Yankee Stadium was as shell-shocked as it ever had been.

"Guess they were due," a chagrined Berra grumbled on the way home that night after watching Boston's Johnny Damon smack two home runs, one a grand slam, in a 10–3 punctuation mark to the first victorious comeback from an 0–3 deficit in baseball's postseason history. From the Yankees' end, payback after so many years was a bitch.

Down in Louisiana, Guidry tried to rationalize what he had seen by raising the possibility that there was more to determining the outcome of a season than runs, hits, and errors. "The good Lord has a way of evening things out," he said. "So you know it's not going to last forever." But even with the world turned upside down, Guidry found himself rooting for the Red Sox in the World Series against the St. Louis Cardinals.

"As much as you have the same feeling that they have for you, when you get to the World Series, I don't pull for the National League. I pull for the American League, even though it was the Red Sox," he said. "Because what you learn as you're going through your career is that people think the National League is better. Well, why are they the better league when the American League has won so many more titles [63–44 after 2011]. You actually get ticked off about the stuff."

Berra happened to like Terry Francona, Boston's rookie manager, whose father, Tito, had played against him in the fifties and sixties. But he took the Yankees collapse hard and wasn't thrilled about his hometown Cardinals getting swept by the Sox.

Back in Tampa the following spring, he told Guidry over dinner that watching the Red Sox beat the Yankees four straight after being down 0–3 and behind in the ninth inning of game four was "like a bad accident where you don't really see it coming, then it hits you, and you wonder what the hell happened."

"Well, yeah," Guidry said. "But they earned it."

"Yeah, maybe they were overdue," Berra agreed.

Guidry could see that Berra was struggling with the altered American League landscape and the concept of the Red Sox as champions and the Yankees as chokers.

"Look at it this way," Guidry told him. "There's nothing against them now the next time they lose, because they actually won. There's no ghost of Babe Ruth, no more curse. You won? Fine, I'm happy for you. Let Babe rest. He has nothing to do with this thing anymore."

Berra nodded. He liked the idea. Finally and forever, the Babe could rest.

8

It Takes a Clubhouse

Ron Guidry needed help. By 2006, he had taken on the full-time position of Yankees pitching coach in addition to his duties as Yogi Berra's social director, and there was only so much time in a spring training day.

Beyond his annual instructor's role, Guidry had never coached, nor had he been eager to leave Lafayette for months on end for any particular job. He had taken this one because Mel Stottlemyre had recommended him and because Joe Torre had asked.

Five years after being diagnosed and successfully treated for multiple myeloma, or cancer of the bone marrow, Stottlemyre was ready to go home to his beloved Washington State. He had always admired Guidry and noticed during past spring trainings how relaxed he was around the pitchers, how well he got along with them.

Bonnie Guidry encouraged Ron to take the job if that's what he wanted to do. So did Berra, who reminded him that he had hired one of Guidry's heroes, Whitey Ford, as his first pitching coach in 1964 while Ford was still pitching.

"Why'd you do that?" Guidry asked.

"Why not?" Berra said. "Whitey was always learning little things that helped him be good. I figured he could teach those things, too. He was never afraid to speak his mind."

Guidry wondered how it worked when pitching coach Ford had to decide whether pitcher Ford should come out of a game. "We talked about it," Berra said. "My first game as manager, Whitey pitched eleven innings. He felt good. Plus Rivera wasn't born then."

Staff closer was one position Guidry didn't have to worry about now, not with the great and seemingly ageless Mo Rivera around. But he did need a crash course in how a contemporary pitching coach went about his work. Being an old-school traditionalist, Guidry didn't really get all the statistical analysis — why, for instance, a pitching coach had to know how to pitch hitter X when it was 74 degrees and partly sunny, as opposed to 50 degrees, overcast, and damp.

Worse, Guidry was electronically challenged. "I don't use a computer, and to be honest, I don't need one to tell me who is good or that this guy hits me well over his career," he said. "It seems like we've been brainwashed into getting so much information."

He found a sympathetic audience in Berra, who loved to tell Guidry and others how in his day, hitters would prepare for a game by taking a few swings — unlike today, when batting practice might turn into a half-day outing in the cage.

Set in his ways, Guidry wound up preparing all of his reports by hand, a time-consuming chore, among others, that left him scrambling to make sure Berra was getting the attention he deserved.

"When he first came back, I'd get up at six thirty every morning, bring him in [to the complex], and I'd be the one to drive him back [to his hotel]," Guidry said. "This went on for years." But now the manager of Berra's itinerary needed his own coaching staff to handle Yogi — a spring training chapter of the Friends of Yogi Inc. Not surprisingly, there was no shortage of volunteers.

The main volunteer was former Yankees manager Carl "Stump" Merrill. As soon as word spread that Yogi Berra was staying at the hotel and that he was routinely in the lobby by 7:00 A.M. sharp, the autograph seekers would gather there every morning, pumped up and ready to pounce. Knowing Berra's punctuality, Merrill would be right there with them, waiting to help his old friend navigate the fans and make his way outside to the car.

"He'd accommodate them, even though they weren't always polite," Merrill said. "But the one thing that bothered him was if he thought they only wanted him to sign something so they could sell it. It's early in the morning, and you think he's just signing his name, but he would look at someone and say, 'I signed for you yesterday.' Oh, he remembers."

Across the road, just a couple of minutes away, Guidry could sleep better knowing that Merrill was with Berra at the hotel. Merrill, he knew, was as loyal to Berra as anyone. In fact, if it hadn't been for Berra, Merrill might never have dressed in a big-league clubhouse.

In June 1981, a strike shuttered the major leagues for fifty days, the first time in baseball history that players walked out during the season. Determined to make his people earn their keep, George Steinbrenner ordered his major-league coaches into the minors to scout and help mentor the organization's prospects. Berra drew Nashville, where Merrill was the manager.

Merrill was a former minor-league catcher with a degree in physical education from the University of Maine. He began working for the Yankees in 1978 at West Haven, Connecticut, in the Eastern League and moved south when the Yankees took control of the Southern League's Nashville team in 1980.

Suddenly, in mid-1981, the former catcher who had never made it out of Double-A ball had the most famous and decorated Yankees backstop asking him, "What do you want me to do?"

Wait a minute, Merrill thought. *Yogi Berra is asking me to supervise him?*

"Do whatever you want," Merrill said.

"No," Berra said. "Give me something specific."

And that was when Merrill began to understand the existential splendor of Yogi Berra, whom he would come to call Lawrence or Sir

Lawrence in comic tribute to his utter lack of pretense and sense of importance.

"He rode buses with us all night," Merrill said. "You think he had to do that? He was incredible."

One day Merrill told him, "Why don't you hit some rollers to that lefty kid over there at first base?"

Berra did as he was told and later remarked to Merrill, "That kid looks pretty good with the glove." Berra knew a prospect when he saw one. It was Don Mattingly, who at the time was considered expendable by a chronically shortsighted organization always on the prowl for immediate assistance at the major-league level.

The Yankees feared that Mattingly would never be strong enough to hold down first base, a power position. Berra was adamant with the brass that when the kid grew stronger, he would have the ability to pull the ball into the friendly right-field porch at Yankee Stadium. When Mattingly became a full-time player under Berra in 1984, he hit .343 with 23 homers and 110 runs batted in. When Mattingly later went on to manage the Dodgers in Los Angeles in 2011, he wore number 8 in tribute to the man who had helped him become a Yankee.

Back in 1981, Merrill learned quickly to appreciate Berra's keen baseball instincts. They became fast friends, and before the 1985 season, Berra asked Merrill to be his first-base coach. Elated, the career minor-leaguer hit the big time, only to watch his friend get unceremoniously canned in Chicago in April and take his storied bus ride with the team to the airport.

"I can still see him standing up and wishing everyone well, with Dale [Berra] sitting right there. Who else does that?" Merrill said, moved by Berra's composure and class.

Merrill lasted only a couple more days himself. In Billy Martin's first game back as manager, the young shortstop Bobby Meacham hit what would have been a three-run home run in Texas — had he not passed Willie Randolph after rounding first. The Yankees lost. Naturally, in the world according to Steinbrenner and Martin, it was Merrill's fault. He returned to the minors to manage at Columbus.

At least Merrill had a job and a title — "organizational lifer." Riding the tides of Yankees change, he coached again with the big team under Lou Piniella, even managing it during the lean years, 1990–1991. In retirement back home in Maine, he would wait for the call every winter inviting him to spring training. He relished the opportunity to pitch in and catch up with his old friend Yogi, whose return to the team had cheered Merrill like no other news.

In the clubhouse, fresh off a good walk on the treadmill, Berra liked to tease Merrill for his ample girth. On the bench, they would reminisce about their days together in Nashville.

"I could never understand why you wanted to sit on those damn buses with us all night," Merrill told him.

"What the heck else was there to do in Nashville?" Berra said.

Merrill knew it was futile to bring up country-and-western music or the fact that Nashville was one of the more entertaining cities in the south. Berra was all business, and his business was baseball.

"He'd be sitting there with guys standing along the rail, and he can barely see the field," Merrill said. "But suddenly he'd say, 'That kid turned the wrong way on the ball,' or 'This guy's got good command.' You think he's just sitting there minding his own business, but it's amazing what he would see."

In the early years of Berra's return to spring training, he and Merrill both stayed at Steinbrenner's hotel. When Steinbrenner sold the place, Guidry invited Berra to come bunk with him in his apartment, an offer he would periodically repeat. "I got the extra bedroom, Yog," he said. "This way we're in the same place."

"It's OK. I'll stay at another hotel," Berra said.

He preferred his independence, especially for when Carmen came into town, and he figured that he was already imposing on Guidry enough. He moved to a nearby Marriott Residence Inn, as did Merrill, with Guidry's blessing.

Berra and Merrill would stay on the same floor, Berra typically in room 108 — "He's got to have an eight in the room number if it's available," Merrill said — with Merrill and his wife, Winnie, right across the hall.

Having Merrill with Berra allowed Guidry to fulfill his more demanding duties as pitching coach. Many mornings, Merrill took over as the designated driver. And while Guidry got his pitchers ready for the games, Berra and Merrill wouldn't waste good weather sitting around the cramped clubhouse or in the dugout. While the players took batting practice, they would walk the outfield warning track, foul pole to foul pole.

"OK, Lawrence, how many we doing today?" Merrill would ask, knowing that Berra would likely choose his favorite number. They would finish the first leg, and Merrill would say, "OK, that's one."

Berra would look at him with a sly grin and say, "You mean two?"

With baseballs flying everywhere, Merrill liked to think of himself as the lookout, since Berra — in his imagined protective bubble — was typically oblivious to the possibility of being struck. "Some people would have said it was the blind leading the blind," Merrill said. "But who was I kidding? The way his life had gone, he could have walked back and forth all by himself, and every ball would somehow miss him."

Merrill was reminded of an old quote that he thought came from the wisecracking ex-Yankee and *Ball Four* author, Jim Bouton: "Yankees die in plane crash; Berra misses flight."

Berra had another volunteer minder in Steve Donohue, the Yankees' assistant trainer and the man personally charged with keeping Berra's neck and shoulders from stiffening up.

"Where you guys going for dinner tonight?" he would ask early in the day, knowing Berra was not one for last-minute scheduling.

"The Rusty Pelican," Berra would say.

"What time?" Donohue knew full well that Berra liked his vodka and dinner at the early-bird hour. Asking was in keeping with the preferred routine.

"Five o'clock."

"Just you and Gator?"

"Yeah, me and Gator."

Donohue would call in the reservation, doing his part in the clockwork organization that Guidry had created to make sure every one of Berra's bases was covered.

There were even occasions when Donohue got the chance to be the driver, mostly on a Sunday morning when Guidry had another commitment and Merrill was off with his wife. "That's when I got called in from the bullpen," he said.

Donohue and Berra also went back a long way — coincidentally, as far back as Merrill and Berra did, to Nashville in 1981. On his way up to the majors, Donohue was the trainer for the Nashville Sounds that year. When Berra came in from New York, they had adjoining hotel rooms.

"He was like all the rest of us," Donohue said. "We used to talk about it — why the hell is this guy sitting with us on the bus for hours? The Southern League was a rough travel league. But being on the bus with us just seemed to make him happy."

On Sunday, Berra wasn't happy until he attended Mass. One Saturday in Tampa, he called Donohue to ask what time they would be going the next day. Donohue said, "Yogi, I've got to get to the ballpark tomorrow to work. What if I find us one for about seven?"

The earlier the better, as far as Berra was concerned. Donohue called back to say he had located a 7:30 Mass on North Himes Avenue. "The good news is that the church is named Saint Lawrence," he said.

Berra was impressed. "No kidding," he said. "I never saw a church named after Saint Lawrence."

They went the next morning. Berra was thrilled, never saying a word about the Mass being in Spanish.

• • •

Of all the Yankees who held Berra near and dear, Joe Torre did the best imitation of him, hands down. Torre, Merrill, and Donohue all inevitably worked an imitation into just about any discussion. Donohue would even occasionally go so far as to converse with Berra in Yogi-speak. Even Guidry gave it a shot, though his Cajun accent did Berra no justice.

But Torre had the knack, the natural ability to lower his voice, contort his face, and bring Berra's sweet grumpiness to life. "Maybe because we're both Italian," he said.

On the subject of his everlasting fondness for Berra, however, Torre was loath to cite their common ethnicity. "I'm not Tommy Lasorda," he said, referring to the former Dodgers manager, who was quick to play the paisano card. "I got to know Yogi when he was coaching for the Mets and I'd come in with the Braves, playing first base. I'd tease him about this or that, and sometimes he took me serious. But it was easy as a player to get close to him because he let you in. What you saw was what you got."

For Torre, that particular term of endearment was never more self-evident than when he had a friend from Hawaii visiting him during spring training. He and the friend were sitting in the manager's office, shooting the breeze, when Torre thought he heard Berra's familiar voice outside in the hall.

"You want to meet Yogi?" Torre asked.

The friend nodded enthusiastically.

"Yogi?" Torre called out. Berra appeared in the doorway, au naturel, not so much as a towel around his waist. He stepped into the room and proceeded to strike up a polite conversation.

"The thing was that Yogi had stepped close to shake my friend's hand, and so now he's standing right in front of the guy, who's sitting down and not knowing where the hell to look," Torre said.

Trying not to burst out laughing, Torre playfully kept the conversation going for as long as he could to extend his friend's discomfort. The guy was continuing to look this way and that way, anywhere but straight in front of him. Torre knew one thing: Berra was not going to excuse himself out of embarrassment. "He has no inhibitions, none whatsoever," Torre said.

This was further illustrated when Berra, Don Zimmer, and Don Mattingly were in the car one day with Torre at the wheel, en route to an away exhibition game. For games that weren't too far from Tampa, Torre and some of the coaches would drive to the games after getting dressed at home.

Along a typical Florida state-route stretch of restaurants and convenience stores, Berra suddenly announced that he had to pee. Torre pulled into the parking lot of a 7-Eleven.

"This OK?" he asked.

"Sure, why not?" Berra said.

He got out and didn't think twice about walking into the place, cleats and all, in his famous pinstriped number 8, Mattingly and Zimmer right behind. "Where's the bathroom?" Berra asked a kid behind the counter, while the jaws of the patrons dropped to the floor.

"Imagine them going home to tell someone, 'Yogi Berra came into the 7-Eleven to take a leak,'" Torre said, still amused by the scene years later. "But, you know, that was all he cared about. He had to go."

With his wife and young daughter joining him in spring training, Torre seldom hung out with the guys, but he knew that part of his job was to circle the date that Berra would be landing in Tampa on his calendar and to prop Berra's golf clubs up against the back wall of his office when they arrived a few days before the man himself. He made sure there was a fresh supply of Ketel One stored safely in the bottom drawer of his desk, as Guidry had recommended, and he reserved a seat next to him in the dugout for Berra. With Zimmer on the other side and Guidry flanking Berra, exhibition games were seldom as tedious as they'd once been.

In his twelve years with the Yankees, Torre never missed a chance to support or comfort Berra. An emotional man not ashamed to cry in tender moments with his team, Torre was right at Berra's side when

Phil Rizzuto died in August 2007 and Berra was summoned by reporters to the dugout for an interview.

Rizzuto had been Berra's closest friend on the Yankees, his "little big brother." They had worked together in the off-season as salesmen in a Newark clothing shop. They had opened a bowling alley — Rizzuto-Berra Lanes in Clifton, New Jersey. Rizzuto was godfather to the Berras' firstborn, Larry.

In the final months of Rizzuto's life, his whereabouts were largely unknown. But Cora Rizzuto gave Berra full visitation privileges to the Green Hill nursing home. Several times a week, he watched movies with his pal, played bingo, even shared an occasional afternoon nip.

Seeing Berra seize up, ready to sob and create a video that would surely go viral on the Internet when someone asked about those visits, Torre put his arm around Yogi and massaged his shoulder. Berra held it together and spoke beautifully about his dear friend, the Scooter.

Ron Guidry's time as pitching coach lasted only two years. In 2008, when Torre was replaced as manager by Joe Girardi, general manager Brian Cashman felt that Guidry had been Torre's hire and wanted Girardi to have a fresh start with his own staff. Guidry suspected the change was coming and accepted it without rancor.

He had enjoyed his time back on the road and in New York, getting to spend more time with his son Brandon, who lives in the city, and, of course, seeing Berra at the stadium. The Yankees failed to reach the World Series in 2006 and 2007, and the coaches took much of the blame — although it was also true that Guidry did not have a championship staff to work with. It was a mix of the aging (Randy Johnson, Mike Mussina, Andy Pettitte) and the inadequate (Kei Igawa, Sidney Ponson). The putative ace was the Taiwanese right-hander Chien-Ming Wang.

Wang won nineteen games both years under Guidry, but as Guidry said, "He never could understand his role as the ace because in the culture he was from, he was taught humility. It was hard for Wang to say, 'I'm the best.'"

For Guidry, losing the job was a case of easy come, easy go. Just as it was when the Yankees made it clear they thought his pitching days were over, no one had to twist his arm to go home to Louisiana. On the way, he turned down Torre's offer to join him in Los Angeles. "I wasn't putting on no Dodgers uniform," he said.

Implicit in that declaration was the fact that changing teams would have taken him away from his best friend, Yogi, during spring training. Instead, Guidry waited for the call to return to the Yankees as a camp instructor.

Upon returning to that role, his first assignment was to prep Girardi for the arrival of Berra, just as he'd done with Torre. Guidry laid out the vodka arrangement, showing Girardi where Torre had kept it, and told him that the golf clubs would be arriving soon, too. Between juggling lineups and getting his team ready for the season, Girardi, who didn't imbibe, stored the Ketel One and kept an eye out to make sure it didn't run dry.

Girardi had already bonded with Berra in 1999 over the perfect game, but now they would spend more time together. No matter who occupied the manager's office, Berra would come in each morning with tidbits of commentary about the previous day's game.

"The big kid looked good last night," he would say of the six-foot-ten pitching prospect Andrew Brackman.

"Cano looks like he's lunging at the ball," he would say of the talented second baseman Robinson Cano.

And because Berra was a man whose life had always been a scripture of routine, there would also have to be room in Girardi's car going to away games.

"He liked to take little catnaps in the car," Girardi said. "But one day we're driving to play the Astros, which is about an hour and fifteen minutes' ride, and we're like ten minutes away and he says, 'You took the wrong way. There's a shortcut. I know there's a shortcut that Torre always took.' So I say, 'OK, I'll get directions for the ride back.' So we're driving back, and it's the exact same way, except we're making all lefts instead of rights. And Yogi says, 'I told you this way was shorter.'"

Joe T. to Joe G. was a seamless transition for Berra. Heck, he thought, they were catchers and Italian — what wasn't to like? Like Torre, Girardi never minded hearing Berra's thoughts about the hardest throwers he had caught, the most challenging pitchers he had worked with, the technique and equipment he had used.

"Yog, how did you catch a guy who threw real hard with that little glove?" Girardi asked.

"I put falsies in there for extra padding," Berra said.

"Falsies? What are you talking about?" said Girardi, who wasn't acquainted with the word.

"You know, the padding from a bra," Berra said, completely baffled that any red-blooded American male didn't know what falsies were.

Generationally, Berra reminded Girardi of his father, Gerald, who had raised five children after the death of his wife when Joe was thirteen. Working as a salesman, a bricklayer, and a bartender, Gerald would do whatever it took to get his kids into college — Northwestern for Joe, the baseball star.

Girardi never for a moment forgot whose sacrifices had gotten him to where he was. After the Yankees won the 1996 World Series, he handed his first championship ring to his father, who wore it proudly as Alzheimer's gradually pulled him into a distant, silent world by the time his son was named manager of the Yankees for the 2008 season. And while nobody replaces a father, having Berra around to plop down on the couch in the office every morning to ask about the kids and other mundane matters helped Girardi maintain a balance.

Seeing Berra with Guidry affirmed Girardi's belief in the power of the Yankees as family and team. "You watch that relationship and the way Gator is with Yogi, and you're proud," Girardi said. "Everybody appreciates having Yogi in spring training, but when you see those two together, the reverence and respect they have, you just get a sense of pride. It's really just like watching a father and a son."

Guidry does not exactly appreciate or agree with the suggestion that he and Berra ever had a father-son relationship. "I mean, I love the old man, but my father's still alive, so I got a father," he said. "It's not like that."

And yet Guidry's voice softened when he reflected on his relationship with Berra, how each year it had grown closer, more special. He felt it deeply, he said, when Larry or Dale would fly into Tampa for a visit and offer to take their father out to dinner or to the ballpark when he had already made plans with Guidry. "That's OK, Gator's got it," Berra would say.

"And when I'd hear that, you don't know how good I felt," Guidry said. "That's why I called him my best friend. The best friend is the guy that you look forward to seeing more than anybody else. And you don't have to be from the same generation to have that. You can be years apart and from two different parts of the world."

For Berra, there was nothing unusual, much less poignant, about the friendship. Oh, he always liked Guidry well enough. But he was never the type to gush with emotion, declare his loyalty or love. Even as a young man, Yogi was no "Huggy Berra."

"Gator, he's a good guy" — that's about as much appreciation as he would express.

It was only natural on Guidry's part to wonder occasionally just what Berra might be thinking. "Sometimes you say to yourself, 'How does he really feel about you?' I catch myself thinking, *Does he really want me doing that?*"

Those who knew Berra best understood the side of him that could come across as demanding and cranky, even self-absorbed. Someone might be doing him a favor, but if it wasn't done the way he expected it to be done — or the way it had been done for him regularly by someone else — he had no problem making his unhappiness known.

Berra once called Dave Kaplan to tell him he wanted to go to Yankee Stadium on a particular Thursday. When Kaplan said, thinking out loud, "Oh, that's my anniversary," Berra didn't say, *Oh, sure, forget it*. He didn't say anything. Kaplan reasoned that his wife, Naomi, would understand and they could celebrate the next day. Then again, it *was* her anniversary. And when Carmen Berra found out that Kaplan had spent his anniversary taking Yogi to the ballpark, she lit into her husband and immediately had an expensive bouquet of flowers sent to the Kaplans' house.

More than anyone, she knew where Yogi was coming from, what he wanted from those closest to him, and, most of all, how much he had given to others. She could recite chapter and verse the times he had opened his arms and his home to friends in need. She remembered especially how he looked after young Yankees such as Bobby Richardson, a shy South Carolinian who had difficulty adjusting to New York City. Yogi was willing to drive him all over town and go out of his way to make sure he was comfortable.

In Berra's playing and coaching days, his home was almost a bed and breakfast for players who needed a place to stay, a good meal, or a swim in the pool. In the late 1970s, the Berras welcomed Mike Ferraro, a journeyman player who had spent time with the Yankees and was hired as a coach. He was trying to save money so that he could keep his home in Fort Lauderdale. Where else to stay but at the Berra B & B?

A decade later, when Berra heard that Ferraro's father had died in Kingston, New York, he drove two hours north and served as a pallbearer at the funeral without Ferraro even asking. Looking back, all Ferraro could say was that he wished that his father, a lifelong Yankees fan, could have gone to his grave knowing that Yogi Berra was going to help carry the casket.

All his life, Berra had done things without being asked and without wanting to be thanked. His intentions were typically rooted in the quest for everlasting camaraderie, normalcy, and simplicity — an escape from celebrity with those disinclined to fawn over him or ask him to autograph their bats.

"The thing is, it's not that hard to get inside his inner circle," said Larry Berra. "Basically, he loves everybody, as long as you are trustworthy and loyal — doesn't matter whether you're the garbage man or the president of the United States."

The person's standing was inconsequential, as long as he or she could make Berra feel comfortable and relaxed and part of his routine. A card-playing buddy could walk by him in the locker room of the Montclair Golf Club and say, "Yogi, I promised myself I'd lose twenty pounds before you die," to which Berra would respond, "Then you better hurry the fuck up." (True story, courtesy of a member who overheard the exchange.)

"People come in and out of Dad's life all the time, but there's not many he has a special trust or affinity for," Dale Berra said. "He can't express it, but you will know if he appreciates you."

His appreciation might come with a nod or a telephone call starting with the greeting, "Whattya doin'?" While those inside the circle seemed to give a lot more than they received, payback for devotion was often a patriarchal belief in them and his trust.

One Father's Day, when asked what he would be doing with the family, Berra said that of course he was going to Yankee Stadium for the game. "That's my family," he rationalized. Harsh as that may have sounded, his family understood.

"Baseball was everything, all we did," Larry Berra said. "That's been his whole life, being around the team and the guys. You either fit in with that or you didn't."

With the exception of his fourteen years away from the Yankees, going to the ballpark had just been part of Berra's day, no more unusual than brushing his teeth. The Yankees were and always would be family, and that was why his sons took no offense to the brushoff they would occasionally get in Tampa: "Gator's got it."

When Larry Berra bunked with his father at the hotel in Tampa, many mornings meant being awakened at the crack of dawn. "Gator's coming to get me," Yogi would say. "You have to get up if you want to come."

Larry would roll over and go back to sleep.

"My attitude was always, *You do what you have to do*," Larry said. *"I got a car. I'll fit in."* He paused for comic effect and added, "But then

I'd tell Gator, 'Don't think you're getting any of the inheritance. You still got to go through me for that.'"

Larry knew Guidry before Yogi did, having played against him in the minor leagues. There was never envy, he said, or perceived threat. Inside the circle, they each knew their place.

At age sixty, Larry moved back in with his parents after a divorce. His job was to make sure that Yogi had his morning papers — "by seven thirty or else," he said — and to be home by eleven on weeknights so that they could watch reruns of *Seinfeld* and *Everybody Loves Raymond*.

"You're late," Berra would growl if Larry plopped down fifteen minutes after eleven.

"Dad, what's the big deal? They'll be showing reruns for the next two hours!"

Larry understood that there was nothing his father hated more than change and surprise. In Tampa, Yogi's time with Guidry and the others was the core of his spring training regimen, and nothing short of an illness or an earthquake could interfere with it. Yes, at times Yogi could be difficult, but his truest and most trusted friends reserved the right to tell him that he was being a royal pain in the ass.

"And if he wants, he can tell me, 'Aw, go to hell,'" Guidry said. "But I think — I hope — it goes deeper than just needing someone to do something. I like to think that he wants *me* doing it, that he's counting on it."

One day while they were on the golf course in Tampa, patiently waiting for the next hole to clear, making small talk about the wind and the way the course was playing, Guidry suddenly felt Berra's meaty hand on his elbow, gripping it tight. Guidry took the gesture not as a way for Yogi to steady himself, but more as a show of affection, a sign of trust, a token of his appreciation.

And the fact of the matter is, Guidry was absolutely right.

9

Ron's Rule

Other than the ballpark, there was no place Yogi Berra preferred to be more during spring training than the golf course with his good friend Gator, two great Yankees left-handers riding around in a cart, cutting each other up.

"Get your butt back over there," Guidry would tell Berra when he strolled toward the seniors' tee before Guidry could strike his ball. He sure as hell wasn't going to risk having to explain to Carmen how her husband's hard head got in the way of his drive.

A longtime golfer, Berra would incessantly remind Guidry of all the shots he *used* to make before age began to weaken his game. Guidry would say, "Yeah, yeah," but he knew that Berra had been pretty good. The man had been playing before Guidry was born.

Not that their levels of competence much mattered when they tossed their clubs into the back of Guidry's truck and slipped away for a round. "It was never about competition, only camaraderie," Guidry said. "Golfing with Yogi was hilarious."

It always is when you get to make up the rules.

If ever there was a game that was unsuited for Berra's wide-ranging and downright unorthodox baseball swing, it should have been the one in which stationary dimpled balls are hit with a much skinnier stick and maddening precision. But Berra not only made golf a life-time passion; he became pretty good at it, too. He had a ten handi-cap through middle age and an excellent short game, all while play-ing — though not putting — *right-handed*.

The switch-golfing business came about one day back in the fifties when Berra, stuck behind a tree, realized he couldn't advance the ball with his lefty club. He borrowed one from a right-handed partner, thrilled himself with a solid drive, and went with the flow from there in a demonstration of ambidexterity and athletic adaptability.

"My father was pretty much good at any game he tried, just kind of a natural because of his hand-eye coordination," Larry Berra said.

Larry remembered Wiffle ball games in the yard with his broth-ers, and his father coming home and demanding a swing. The boys would scream that he was standing too close to the pitcher and that he'd never make contact. The next thing they knew, the ball would be gone, over the roof and lost in the bushes.

"He was like that with golf, too," Larry said. "He'd hit all these trick shots, and the one place you never wanted to be was one stroke ahead of him with two holes to go. He'd play around with you — 'Watch this. I'm gonna hit this ball within five feet of the hole.' And then he would, no big deal."

Berra was no stage or zealous sports parent, but golf outings with his sons were destined to end up in a shouting match. "You'd miss a short putt, and he'd bark at you, 'How the hell can you miss that?'" Larry said. "He just was born to compete, and he couldn't keep quiet. But in the end, it was all for fun."

Berra took up golf early in his baseball career, before relocating to New Jersey year-round. He played in St. Louis with the likes of Stan Musial, Red Schoendienst, and his childhood idol, Joe Medwick. He loved to play during spring training when the Yankees were based in St. Petersburg, at least until Casey Stengel ordered the clubs put away by the start of the season.

"Pack 'em up," Stengel would say back in the days when managers could get away with such authoritarianism, "and if we catch you out there playing golf, it will cost you two hundred bucks."

As Berra noted, "Two hundred bucks was a lot of money back then."

Fellow catcher and Hall of Famer Al Lopez had recommended the game, telling him, "Play as long as you can. It'll keep you young and healthy." Lopez meant psychologically more than physically, although who's to say how much the two are related?

When Berra's knee deteriorated in his midseventies, he cited golf as the main reason to go through the trauma of replacement and rehabilitation. By then the game had become too central to his life to let a little surgery get in the way.

"Why wouldn't you?" he reasoned. "I always liked to play. It's a nice way to spend the day. You get exercise, fresh air, competition."

Over the years, golf also gave him an excuse to travel. He played in charity events all over the country, doing old baseball buddies a favor in the process. Berra went all the way to North Dakota to appear in Roger Maris's tournament, to Oklahoma City for the former Yankees pitcher Ralph Terry, and to Florida for Whitey Ford, to name just a few.

He became a regular at the Bob Hope Classic, a main PGA Tour event in the Southern California desert. The comedian, who died at age one hundred in 2003, had gotten to know Berra when he had a stake in the Cleveland Indians and began inviting him to his January tour event in the midnineties — a good excuse for Berra to escape the New Jersey winter. Eventually, the organizers made him the classic's first ambassador, and he continued to show up for the celebrity pro-am there years after Hope's death.

In an extension of his minimalist approach to batting practice, Berra took few, if any, practice shots while playing in the Hope Classic. "I know what I have to do," he would say, always worried about cluttering his head with too much analysis of his swing.

Rene Lagasi, a retired pharmaceutical manager and a New Jersey friend and neighbor, was his frequent golf companion and caddy in the Hope Classic. Lagasi had a home in the desert, where he would host Berra and accompany him to breakfast—Berra would go off diet to satisfy a craving for an Egg McMuffin at McDonald's—before heading off to the golf course.

Berra often managed to say something that would help keep a good walk comical and unspoiled.

One day while Berra was playing in a foursome that included Lagasi and Johnny Lujack, the former Notre Dame quarterback and 1947 Heisman Trophy winner, all four players hit their balls on the green not far apart. When they approached the green, Lujack asked, "Yogi, where are you?" Berra replied, "I'm right here."

Faced once with a difficult lie, he complained to a partner that his shot was likely to end up in the water. "Yogi, don't think like that; think positively," his partner said. "OK," he decided. "I'm positive my shot is going into the water."

Out of thin air, he would coin a mathematical aphorism and instant Yogi-ism, declaring once, "Ninety percent of short putts don't go in."

For Berra, golf represented a diversion from baseball, but somehow it had a way of intersecting with the game. He was on a New Jersey golf course after the 1954 season, waiting out a cloudburst, when he received the news that he had been named the American League's most valuable player for the second time. He immediately got a champagne toast from his companions.

He once negotiated a contract with Yankees owner Dan Topping over eighteen holes, cleverly asking Topping what he thought his star catcher was worth. Berra liked the answer and said, "You got a deal." In the process, Berra circumvented the stubborn general manager, George Weiss, with whom he regularly had contract squabbles. Weiss was furious when he found out, barking at Topping, "*You* can sign them from now on."

The job news he received at the country club wasn't always so uplifting, however. Berra was on the course the day after sending Mel Stottlemyre out to lose game seven of the 1964 World Series when he got word that the Yankees wanted to see him in the office the next day. He crossed the bridge into the Bronx, expecting a contract extension, and returned to New Jersey with his walking papers.

In 1972, on the worst day of his long golfing life, Berra and the rest of Gil Hodges's Mets coaching staff were playing eighteen holes near the end of spring training. Walking back to his hotel, Hodges collapsed and died of a massive heart attack. Berra was named manager days later in the saddest appointment of his career.

On the whole, golf for Berra was eminently good because it connected him with people and allowed him to continue to feel vital long after his retirement from baseball. In 1991, he started his annual charity golf tournament to benefit special needs children, and eventually the event became the primary fundraiser for his museum's educational programs.

It was at his own tournament that Berra notched the only hole in one of his life. He didn't count it, because by then he had taken to playing host by stationing himself at the eighth hole and hitting a couple of tee shots with each group as they passed through. "I hit enough balls," he said, "and one went in."

One of his favorite days each year was when he got to stand in front of the Montclair Golf Club on the morning of check-in, welcoming Yankees past and present as they arrived, lugging their clubs through the parking lot and into the locker room. Many of the players lived in the area, but a few would fly in for the event, an all-day affair that concluded with an evening dinner.

After his retirement, Mel Stottlemyre flew across the country several times from his home in Washington State to play in the tournament. Joe Torre usually made it his business to show up (and Berra reciprocated by playing in Torre's tournament). But as his relationship with Guidry evolved, it was Guidry for whom he waited anxiously, badgering Dave Kaplan and others for news of his arrival from Louisiana.

Guidry would arrange for an autograph show or two in the New York area around the time of the tournament and spend some time with his son. But he knew that Berra wanted him there. Across the decades, Berra had golfed with everyone from the rocker Alice Cooper to the legend Arnold Palmer to Presidents George Bush (squared), Bill Clinton, and Gerald Ford. But Guidry had become his favorite partner in the years since time had taken its inevitable toll on his game. Putting became a challenge, and reaching the green could be a multistroke misadventure. Lamenting his lack of driving power, Berra said, "I hit a baseball farther than I do a golf ball now."

For a man long used to competing with pride and triumphing over doubts about his physical capabilities, golf had the potential to become the most humbling and embarrassing experience of all. But that never happened when Berra played a round of eighteen in Tampa after a day at the ballpark. Not on Ron Guidry's watch, at least.

Guidry was almost fifty years old when Berra returned to the Yankees in the spring of 2000. He had been golfing for ten years, having taken the game up after retiring from baseball. Good at every sport he ever tried, Guidry picked up this one without great difficulty, playing with a handicap as low as six when he was firing on all cylinders.

"I'm always around eighty/eighty-one, but I can get it down to seventy-seven or seventy-eight when I'm really playing a lot," he said. "There's always that one hole on the course where I end up with a double bogey, triple bogey, but I'll shoot eighty/eighty-one pretty normally."

Not that his score much mattered to him as the years passed. In the arena of athletic combat, Guidry was a man at peace, mostly with himself. Whatever he needed to achieve he had already done so throwing fastballs and sliders. He didn't need the stress of trying to prove anything. On the golf course, the social and recreational benefits were all he was seeking to accrue.

At home in Lafayette, Guidry had a regular game with a friend, another left-hander. They met every Tuesday morning at eight o'clock sharp for eighteen holes. In a couple of cathartic hours, riding around in a cart, they didn't bother with pencils, scorecards, or the emotional baggage of blowing a hole.

"Most of the time when I'm playing, that's how it is," he said. "I don't worry about the score. Where am I going, to the senior tour? What's a handicap going to do for me at this point? Golf is a great sport to play, but it's just for enjoyment, for peace of mind. It's great to just get on a course, whack the ball, and get your frustrations out."

That made Guidry the perfect partner for Berra, who was seventy-four when he returned to spring training in 2000 and was rarely able to break a hundred on the course. Oh, he could still hit the ball solidly and occasionally drive it a fair distance — enough to inspire Guidry to think, *I hope I can hold a golf club in my hands and do that for as long as he has.*

But it didn't take long for Guidry also to see that the golf course could become cruel to the elderly and that Berra — notwithstanding his athletic pedigree and excellent conditioning for a man his age — was no exception.

"He gets to a par five that's about six hundred yards long, and even though he's hitting from the seniors' tee, it's going to take him at least five shots to even get close enough to the green, much less have a chance to make par," Guidry said. "Now, on a par four, which might be only about three hundred fifty yards, he's starting from the seniors' tee, so now all he's got to go is about three hundred ten. OK, he might smack two great shots, and then he's right off the green. But he still has to get there and then get the ball to the hole."

Scorecard or no scorecard, Guidry could tell from the first time they played that Berra, still driving himself to compete, was increasingly frustrated by how long it took him to finish a hole. Guidry also knew that the courses weren't getting any shorter and that Berra wasn't getting any younger. Something had to give, because he knew for damn sure that stubborn ol' Yogi wasn't about to give up.

• • •

Before going out to play eighteen holes, Guidry asked the General to step over to the side, out of Berra's earshot. "I want you to know that I got only one rule on the golf course that I need you to play by," he said.

"OK, no problem, what is it?" the General said.

"You'll see when we get out on the course," Guidry said.

The General wondered what the heck Guidry could be talking about but figured he would find out soon enough.

Most colleagues and friends knew Brigadier General Arthur F. Diehl III by his nickname, "Chip," but to Guidry and Berra he was just "the General." They had met him at Legends Field in Tampa (before it was renamed for George Steinbrenner) when Diehl had been invited by Steinbrenner to throw out the first pitch of a Yankees spring training game, with a coordinated military flyover.

Forever proud of making second lieutenant in the Air Force before an honorable discharge in 1954, Steinbrenner tended to celebrate all things military and especially its leaders. In the Boss's mind, there was no bigger hero in the Tampa Bay area in the years after September 11, 2001, than Chip Diehl, commander of MacDill Air Force Base, four miles southwest of downtown Tampa.

On 9/11, Diehl was working in Washington at the Pentagon when American Airlines flight 77 was hijacked out of Dulles International Airport by five al-Qaeda terrorists and flown into the western section of the building, killing all 64 people aboard and 125 people inside. His office was on the opposite side, near the river entrance. "You could feel the whole building shake," he said.

With the country knocked far off its foundation, Diehl was soon after assigned by General Tommy Franks at Central Command to mobilize the coalition of countries in support of the Bush administration's global war on terror. To begin the operation, he was sent to MacDill, which meant going home: Diehl had been born on the base when his father, an Air Force pilot, was stationed there in the late fifties and on through the Cuban missile crisis in 1962.

On the day he threw out the first pitch at Legends Field, Diehl met Joe Torre and took the opportunity to mention the two golf courses on the base. He invited Torre and friends to come play when they had a chance.

Torre took him up on the offer, calling later to ask if he could bring a group over. "Are you kidding? We'd love to have you," Diehl said. The next day, Torre, Don Zimmer, Reggie Jackson, Don Mattingly, Berra, and Guidry rode over and made one request — that Diehl play with them. He joined a foursome with Guidry and Berra.

The first hole was a straightaway par three, and right away Guidry gave the General a feel for how entertaining the afternoon would be.

"Where the hell are you going?" Guidry said when Berra got out of the cart and began walking in the direction of the seniors' tee.

"To hit my shot," Berra said.

"Are you kidding me?" Guidry said. "You want one of us to whack you in the back of the head with our ball? You're shooting last."

Diehl wondered, *Could this be the rule that Guidry was talking about?*

It wasn't. But he found out soon enough what it was after Berra put his tee shot straight down the middle of the fairway, hit a second shot that left him within striking distance of the green, and hit a third that plopped down on the edge, though still a considerable distance from the cup.

"That's good," Guidry yelled. "That's par."

He turned to Diehl and said, "If he gets on the green, he don't putt. That's my rule."

Diehl just watched as Berra obediently walked over to the ball, picked it up, and dropped it into his pocket.

When Diehl or anyone else asked Guidry why Berra didn't have to putt, he shook his head. "I don't have to explain my ideas," he said. "He just doesn't have to."

Diehl, for one, didn't need it spelled out for him. He understood perfectly what Guidry was doing. "He never wanted Yogi to feel embarrassed about how many shots he might need or anyone they played with to get frustrated with the pace," Diehl said. "And he wasn't going to talk about it because he didn't want anyone to misunderstand why he was doing it. It wasn't a function of limitation. It was purely out of respect and to make sure that this will be another day that Yogi goes out and has a good time."

Diehl is an observant man. His military background ensures that he pays close attention to detail. That first time he hosted the Yankees at MacDill, he noticed something about the group over lunch that he found familiarly heartening.

Berra was seated to his right, though not at the head of the table. The rest of the Yankees all had their chairs turned in Berra's direction. Diehl's immediate observation was that it was not a coincidence.

"I said [to myself], 'Hmm, isn't this interesting?'" he said. "And the next time they came out, Yogi wasn't with them but Torre was, and it was the same thing. All the chairs were contoured toward Joe."

Diehl was enough of a baseball fan — he had family in Philadelphia and had rooted for the Phillies growing up, while paying proper homage to the Yankees of the early 1960s — to know that New York's success was at least partly predicated on its vast financial resources. But there was something more about this team that he would not have known had he not seen it at close range.

It was, Diehl said, a chain of command that was more than adhered to; it was expected and appreciated. He could see the effects of it at the dinner table or when he brought a friend to a game in Tampa and several players signed a ball for him, intuitively leaving the sweet spot vacant for manager Joe Girardi, who signed it there last.

Most of all, he marveled at how attentive Guidry was to Berra, how enthusiastically he took on the responsibility, and how seriously he went about making sure Berra was comfortable and happy.

"You grow up with beliefs about certain famous people," Diehl said. "For me, Yogi Berra was more than a baseball icon. He represented the best of America, the values that say you can succeed no matter what your background is and no matter how many people say you can't. When I saw how devoted Gator was to Yogi, how much he honored what Yogi had meant not only to him but everyone else, it affirmed those beliefs. I saw their relationship through a military aperture: *You were there for me. I don't care how old you are. I'm going to take care of you.*"

Guidry impressed Diehl as the ultimate teammate, the guy you'd want with you in a foxhole or flying alongside you into battle. Over time, they developed a friendship that was closer than any Diehl had with the other Yankees. It also went well beyond golf. He visited Guidry in Louisiana, staying at his home, meeting his parents, hitting the links around Lafayette.

Back in Tampa, Guidry — often with Berra — became the most regular visitor to the base for a round with the General, who was only three years younger than Guidry. Although Guidry had served in the National Guard, it was Berra, a World War II veteran and part of the naval invasion of Normandy in June 1944, who had old war stories to share.

"They got to be good friends, Yogi and the General," Guidry said. "So there'd be a lot of times that we'd play that I'd get Yogi to ride with him. Yogi was tickled to death. I figured they were both in the military. Let them talk."

Berra filled Diehl in on his history. He was a gunner's mate aboard the USS *Bayfield,* which was the flagship for the invasion force landing at Utah Beach. He wound up as one of a six-man crew on a thirty-six-foot-long rocket boat, going in first, running interference and targeting German bunkers on the bluffs in front of the first landing craft carrying the assault waves of troops.

Berra was eighteen, curious, and somewhat oblivious. He told Diehl that as the sky lit up with explosions, he took a moment from helping loading the rocket launcher to admire the view, which reminded him of the Fourth of July. That got his officer's attention. "You better get your head down if you want to keep it on," he barked.

Diehl said that Berra was more sheepish about another experience, three days before D-day, when he and his mates floated out in the rocket boat to watch for low-flying planes. When one appeared below the clouds, they followed orders and shot it down, forcing the pilot to eject. Unfortunately, the plane, which crashed in the water not far from the boat, was American.

"Boy, that pilot was ticked," Berra told Diehl. "But, you know, those were our orders."

"Sounds right," said Diehl, who sensed that Berra wasn't sure he was convinced that they had not been negligent.

"Yogi, I believe you," he said.

"OK, good," Berra said.

Hearing Berra talk about his wartime experiences with such enthusiasm gave Diehl an idea. He arranged for a foursome — the three of them and another World War II veteran named Willie O'Donnell, who was a few years older than Berra and had flown B-25 bombers over Europe. "Every time we turned around, they were in the cart, telling their old war stories," Diehl said. "We got such a kick out of it. And afterward, Willie says to me, 'Yogi Berra. He was like every other regular guy I knew over there.'"

In the months and years after the invasions of Afghanistan and then Iraq, Guidry or Berra would occasionally shoot a question or two at Diehl about his work in the war on terror. Sometimes he would answer. Other times he would say, "Uh, let's change the subject." They knew not to press the issue or to be insulted when Diehl's office would cancel a golf date at the last minute. "That's when he was in command, and things were pretty heavy," Guidry said.

Diehl retired from the military in 2005, although he continued to make an occasional trip to Afghanistan or Iraq to consult or help with the ongoing operations. A couple of times, he brought back keepsakes for Guidry and Berra — foreign currency, a flag from one of the countries with forces in the area, a hat commonly worn in local culture. Guidry called the General "a jewel of a person, the kind of guy you love spending a few hours with on the golf course, because he could really appreciate all the little things."

One day Diehl brought a friend named Roger to fill out the foursome. Roger, a baseball fan, proceeded to wilt under the pressure of playing with the famous Berra and Guidry. It was a hacker's nightmare, one hole after another. In the middle of the round, Roger hit a ball into the bunker and looked like he was going to cry.

Diehl felt terrible for him and wanted to do something to cheer him up. "Roger," he said, "it's not so bad. Look over there." In the distance, Berra was hard at work in the sand trap, smoothing it over for Roger to hit his way out.

"Yogi, you don't have to do that," Roger yelled, mortified.

"No," Berra said, "that's OK."

Diehl patted his friend on the back and told him, "Keep it in perspective. It's not every day that you turn around and see Yogi Berra raking the sand trap for you, is it?"

The General knew the difference between a golf course and a war zone. He recognized the beauty of competition without obsessive scorekeeping and the benefits of helping even the oldest folks to feel young. The longer he played by the Guidry rule, the more he asserted himself in enforcing it.

"It got to the point with the General that when Yogi would get on the green, I wouldn't have to say a thing," Guidry said. "He'd be riding with Yogi, and I would be with whoever the other guy was, and the General would point to Yogi's ball and say, 'That's good. You're done.' And then he'd turn to the other guy — it could be a major from the base, a colonel, whatever — and say, 'You've got to put yours in.'"

Guidry was delighted to relinquish the reins. He had the General well trained, and nobody, least of all Berra, was going to argue with the base commander.

10

Frog Legs and Friends

The first harbinger of spring — or spring training — at the home of Ron and Bonnie Guidry was a telephone call from Yogi Berra.

"You get the frog legs yet?" Berra would ask.

"Yog," Ron Guidry would say, "it's freaking January."

Too late, Berra was already in serious countdown mode for the next Guidry frog fry extravaganza.

It seemed like only yesterday that Berra had looked askance at Guidry's beloved delicacy, like it was tofu wrapped in seaweed. It had actually been years since Mel Stottlemyre had bragged one spring training day about hunting frogs in the Northwest and cooking them himself. Guidry, with all due respect, was obliged to inform him that he hadn't really experienced frog legs until he'd had them Cajun-style, or straight from the Guidry family cookbook.

Guidry returned to his apartment that evening, fried up a fresh batch, and the next day passed them around the coaches' room. He offered one to Berra, who immediately made a face.

"Come on," Guidry said. "You'll like 'em."

Stottlemyre, munching nearby, couldn't disagree. But still Berra demurred.

"Yogi, I'll tell you what, if you don't try one, we're not going to supper tonight," Guidry said.

Was he serious? Probably not, but if Berra knew one thing about Guidry, it was that he was proud of his Cajun culture and cuisine. Yogi wondered if he was in some way hurting his friend's feelings.

So he finally gave in, picked one off the plate, and gave it a nibble. Lo and behold, it was delicious. He wanted another, and as the years rolled by, he would continue to find a place in his diet for something no conscientious doctor would have ordered for a man in his eighties.

Following treatment in the seventies for an arrhythmia, Berra assiduously watched what he ate. He avoided cholesterol-heavy breakfasts, pushed away most desserts with a dismissive "too fattening," and made sure that the Progresso soup prepared for him at his museum almost daily and specifically at noon by the museum's faithful business manager Bettylou O'Dell was low in sodium.

He had even long ago disassociated himself from the Yoo-hoo soft drink that he had made famous in the fifties and sixties (by chiming in a commercial, "Me-he for Yoo-hoo!") because he objected to the preservatives that had changed the drink's texture and flavor.

If he relaxed his calorie counting, it was usually at dinner, especially at big family dinners, where everyone down to the youngest of the Berras was taught that the heels of the long Italian bread were reserved for Grandpa. Berra's favorite dish was tripe — the stomach tissue of cows and a peasant staple in the old country — but he enjoyed a fairly wide range of gastronomic fare that occasionally didn't agree with him.

For instance, he liked to munch on hot peppers right out of the jar. It was another habit that Carmen wanted him to break — except it turned out that Guidry, who used peppers to spice up his Cajun cooking, was Berra's main supplier.

"I'd have them with me in spring training, and then when he'd go back to New Jersey, he'd tell me to send him a batch when I got back to Louisiana," Guidry said. When Guidry would comply, he would get a call from Carmen asking that he stop sending the peppers. When he didn't send them the next time Yogi asked, he'd get a call wanting to know where the peppers were. "Either way, I had one of them fussin' about the damn peppers," he said with mock resignation.

After so many years of sitting across the table from him at one Tampa establishment or another, Guidry could probably expound on Berra's culinary preferences better than anyone but Carmen. At the very least, he could discuss them like a comedian working his monologue.

"When we go to the Rusty Pelican, that's a seafood place and they have swordfish, which he loves, so he gets that all the time there," Guidry said. "When we go to the Bahama Breeze, he likes the black bean soup, and with that he'll have the seafood paella or the barbecued ribs. Four times out of five, he'll have the seafood, but let's say we have been to the Pelican the night before, well, that means he's already had seafood, so he'll get the ribs.

"Now Fleming's is the steakhouse, so that's what he gets there, and then at the Bonefish he has to have the sea bass. Then after he moved into the Residence Inn, he went one night to eat with Carmen at Lee Roy Selmon's, which is right next door. So he tells me the next day, 'Hey, it's not bad.' The guy recognized him, sat him at a nice table, everything was fine. OK, so now we got to go to Selmon's, and there he gets the meatloaf. But since he's been at the Residence Inn, where they put out a spread in the evening, he also keeps a list on the door of his refrigerator that tells him what they'll be serving. If he likes something he's had before, he'll say, 'On Tuesday, I'm going to eat in the hotel.' 'OK, that's good, Yog.'"

No Tampa meal, however, was as anticipated and as fussed over as Guidry and Berra's "Frog Legs Night," which by the end of Berra's first decade back with the Yankees had taken on the ritualistic weight of Old-Timers' Day.

Before leaving for Tampa every spring, and after being badgered by Berra, Guidry would pack about two hundred legs into the truck, having purchased them inexpensively (about $200 for a hundred pounds) in Lafayette, where they are plentiful and sold year-round. From the same vendor, he would buy a mixture of flour and cornmeal seasoning in a gallon jar.

"They're so simple to fix," Guidry said. "You got the egg batter, the fry mix, dip 'em in the batter, throw 'em in the frying pan." From the frying pan, the frog legs would be transferred to paper towels, to soak up some of the grease. It took about ten minutes to cook up a batch of forty legs.

Guidry would ration his supply so that it would last throughout spring training. He would prepare some for the more adventurous players looking for a break from the standard clubhouse fare. Jorge Posada was a longtime fan. CC Sabathia joined the club when he came on board in 2009. Guidry would also invite two or three buddies over on one of his first nights in town and playfully have Goose Gossage dial New Jersey to let Berra know what was on the menu that night.

"Yogi, we're over here at Gator's, and we're eating all the frog legs," Gossage would say.

That was enough to set Berra off. "There'd better be some goddamn legs left when I get down there," he'd growl.

Guidry was way ahead of him, having set aside enough for Berra's Frog Legs Night, knowing that he was good for about eight or nine, accompanied by sides of sweet potato and green beans wrapped in bacon. If they were eating in, Berra wasn't settling for a snack.

"Everything's got to be just the way it was the last time and the time before that," Guidry said. "If I forget one thing, he'll look at the plate and say, 'Where the *hell* is the sweet potato?'"

Berra would choose the night, usually in March and timed to an NCAA tournament basketball game he was eager to watch. A wide-ranging sports fan, he enjoyed March Madness and happened to be a devout follower of the Rutgers University women's team, coached by C. Vivian Stringer — who once offered him a seat on the bench for a game when she learned he was a Scarlet Knights fan.

"If Rutgers was playing, that was a good night for the frog legs," said Steve Donohue, the rare person allowed into Guidry's place when he was cooking for Berra.

Berra protected the occasion as he would his wallet, typically limiting the guest list to Donohue. In Cooperstown for the Hall of Fame's induction weekend one summer, Kevin McLaughlin, a family friend who had been accompanying Berra to autograph signings for more than twenty years, said he had heard about Guidry's frog legs dinners and wondered if he might be able to arrange an invitation for the following spring. Guidry pointed to Berra and said, "You'll have to ask *him*."

"No," Berra said. He might have been kidding — but probably not.

Donohue was included because he was part of the inner Tampa circle — a dedicated masseur, a trusted colleague, a Yankees lifer — and, well, because Berra needed *someone* to drive him the short distance to Guidry's apartment without having to take the chef away from his work.

"Most of the guys in Tampa, you look in their refrigerator, and you'll see a bottle of water and a loaf of bread," Donohue said. "Gator's got the whole kitchen set up — the pots, the pans — and whenever he would cook the frog legs, you could see how serious he was."

For Guidry, cooking had long been as earnest an undertaking as pitching. He learned to appreciate the subtleties of the art — the same way he could distinguish the movement on a four-seam fastball compared to a two-seamer. To the common assertion that frog legs are pretty much the same delicacy as chicken wings, he would scoff, "That's a dirty-ass bird. Frog legs are much better."

Thrilled with the taste, Berra would nod in full and devoted agreement. It was his own way of recognizing the pride Guidry had in his cooking and the satisfaction he derived from sharing it.

"They're his specialty, and Gator goes all out," Berra said. "It's like watching one of those famous chefs."

But chefs, like coaches, are evaluated on performance and are subject to being replaced when the restaurant changes hands. When

Guidry was let go as pitching coach at the start of the Joe Girardi regime, and with George Steinbrenner fading as a presence in the operation of the ball club, there was really no guarantee that Guidry would be invited back as a spring training instructor.

The uncertainty weighed on Berra throughout the off-season. Left to wonder, he could do only one thing: call Guidry during the winter, early and often.

Did you get the frog legs yet?

It was Berra's way of finding out what he needed to know without asking the more sensitive question. If Guidry had made the purchase, didn't that mean he was planning to be back in Tampa and at the airport to pick Berra up when he arrived?

Guidry would roll his eyes, tell him to calm down, and hang up the phone with a smile fit for spring. He knew exactly what Berra meant. And that, he said, felt good.

Only once did Berra agree to a large frog legs gathering, but that was in New Jersey on the night before his 2010 golf tournament.

Before the annual event, Carmen and Yogi would host a dinner at their Montclair home for those visiting from out of town. After hearing Berra rave about the frog legs for years, Carmen suggested that Guidry bring a batch with him and prepare them in her kitchen.

He agreed on one condition: he would do all the cooking and cleanup. She had to promise not to lift a finger or to so much as wash a single pot or pan.

But after all she had heard, Carmen, a proud cook in her own right, was curious to know just how Guidry went about preparing his famous frog legs. She asked if she could at least observe.

"Carm, leave him alone," Yogi said, pleading with her to give the maestro his space.

Guidry waved him off. "She can stay," he said. "You get your butt in there with everyone else."

Berra shrugged and went off to talk baseball with Goose Gossage and Graig Nettles. When Carmen asked if she could help, Guidry put her to work on the stove, operating the gauges. She was amazed by his confidence in her kitchen, the way he made it his own.

"I told you, Carm," Berra said when dinner was served.

Those were his last words until he had polished off half a dozen legs.

When the golf outing was rained out the next day, Carmen consoled her disappointed husband by reminding him that he had been fortunate to have experienced a taste of spring training in Montclair.

Berra had never visited the Guidrys in Louisiana, and given the passage of years and his advancing age, he probably never would. Guidry understood, of course, but part of him was disappointed that Berra would never see for himself that the "swamp" is actually a pretty sweet place to live.

Most of all, Guidry would have loved for Yogi and Carmen to come down to stay with him and Bonnie and to spend some quality time with his parents. Accents aside, he believed they would find much common ground in their stubborn but transcendently sincere approaches to life.

"My dad was hard-working, but I can never remember him really giving me a whip—my momma, yes, but not my dad," he said. "My dad was just set in his ways, a little like Yogi, and there were times he just wasn't going to be happy. But as much as you wanted to strangle him sometimes when you were growing up—you know, the conflict between parents and kids—you get to a point when you realize, well, I know what you were trying to teach me. I finally get that, because now I have kids and they're doing the same things.

"My dad, he doesn't say much. I mean, he knows how much we love him, and I know that he's proud of me because I turned out to be an OK kid. And I do think he feels an appreciation for the way I look at Yogi. He knows Yogi is not going to take his place, so I think he can appreciate that it's all because of the way he and Momma brought me up — that this is the way I should be treating the guy that meant so much to me in my career.'"

In the Guidry home, gratitude has always been expressed in the kitchen, and Guidry learned from his father that it is perfectly acceptable for a man to have a place there. More than a hobby, cooking has been a passion for Rags Guidry, a source of existential pride. Cajuns, he believes, can in large part be defined by food.

Two of his favorite sayings: "A Cajun is a man of great friendliness who will give you the crawfish off his table" and "Little Cajun children are made of gumbo, boudin, sauce piquant, crawfish stew, and *oreilles de cochon* [pig's ear pastries]."

Over the years, Rags Guidry had devoted so much time and energy to culinary endeavors that he finally decided to put them into printed form, self-publishing a one-hundred-page booklet of recipes — his own and those of family members and friends, including his famous son. He called it *Rags Guidry's Cajun Cookbook* and spiced it with delightful archetypal homilies, tender commentary, and even a touch of political cynicism.

For example, under the heading "Rags's Mother's Depression Era Boiled Eggs and Dried Shrimp Gumbo," he wrote:

> Since fresh shrimp were not generally available where we lived during the Depression, everyone would use dried shrimp. Times were tough, thanks to the Republican Party. My father was a tenant farmer. We raised ducks, turkeys, hogs, sheep, cattle and especially chickens. I remember every four or five days walking about two miles with a basket of two-to-three dozen eggs to sell at the country store. He would pay us 12 cents a dozen. I could buy a pack of dried shrimp for about three cents and it contained more shrimp than you can get today for $2.

The booklet contains page after page of intricate recipes — Rags's Cajun Blackbird Jambalaya, Cajun Italian Meat Loaf, Bacon-Wrapped

Chicken Gizzard, Rags's *special* vegetable soup, his *favorite* sweet potato pie, his chef salad à la Rags.

Mixed among the recipes are photos of a much younger Ron demonstrating the art of cleaning crawfish and of Bonnie demonstrating how to prepare a roux and crawfish gumbo. There are dishes solely devoted to Travis Guidry — his preferred meals on designated nights. There are several variations of frog legs, including frog legs smothered, frog legs court bouillon, and Ron's real fried Cajun frog legs.

The index in the back lists Rags's, Ron's, and Bonnie's recipes in separate categories. Ron is credited with six different rabbit dishes — though it was a rabbit stew prepared by his father in the late seventies that attracted the attention and appetite of no less a critic than George Steinbrenner himself.

Back then the Boss had forged his own Louisiana connection — a close relationship with Eddie Robinson, the legendary football coach at Grambling State University. In 1970, Yankee Stadium hosted the inaugural Whitney M. Young Jr. Memorial Classic, a football game between two historically black colleges, one of which was often Grambling. Steinbrenner went a step further in the spring of 1977 by sending his American League–champion Yankees to the Grambling campus for the first of several charity exhibitions, presenting Rags and Grace Guidry with the perfect opportunity to take Travis on a two-hour road trip to see his brother.

"Do you want me to bring the team some home cooking?" Rags asked Ron one year.

"Drinking and eating, you know, that's always a priority over here," Ron told him.

So the Guidrys rolled into Grambling early, located the baseball field, set up shop under a big shade tree, and went to work. When the team bus pulled in, Ron greeted his family and gave his father the game plan: everyone would be introduced to the crowd prior to the game; most of the regulars would play a couple of innings; after a shower, they'd be ready to eat.

When Ron was done on the field, he went out by the tree and took a seat in the shade. From there he could see Steinbrenner walking around near the Yankees' dugout, looking all distracted. "I knew he could smell the aroma—it was like, what the heck *is* that?" Guidry said. "All of a sudden, he sees us and starts walking over. I'm thinking, *Uh-oh.*"

"Is there a problem?" Rags asked his son.

"We're about to find out," Ron said.

Steinbrenner, however, was smiling and apparently hungry. After being introduced to Guidry's parents, he said, "Whatever you're cooking smells good."

"I'm cooking rabbits, Ronnie's favorite," Rags said. "Why don't you sit down and try some?" Steinbrenner found himself a spot and spent half an hour chowing down on the stew and chatting up the Guidry family.

"And that's how it all started with him," Ron said. "At the end of every season, he'd tell me, 'Don't plan on coming to spring training unless you come with some rabbit.' Every year I'd cook and freeze 'em and bring 'em with me."

Year after year, long beyond his playing days, when Guidry would run into Steinbrenner for the first time in spring training, the Boss would shake his hand, ask how Bonnie and the kids were doing, and then inquire about the rabbit stew. "I got it," Guidry would say, promising to prepare it for the first night game, provided the Boss would be in attendance.

"Oh, I'll be here," Steinbrenner would assure him. On the appointed night, he would wait in his box for Guidry to bring him an extra-large portion of stew.

Before long, the routine had become another Yankees rite of spring.

If Steinbrenner got the benefit of the rabbit stew, Ron Guidry arrived in New York for the 2011 Old-Timers' Day with the ultimate gift for his frog-legs-loving pal. But it was a gift from Rags, not Ron, a copy of the family cookbook with a special insert on page two. Rags Guidry wrote:

This is a personal copy of my Cajun recipes and the first off the press. Some (of the recipes) have been copied with the permission of the persons supplying the recipes; some are of my own creation; some have been hand-me-downs. I know that you may not try all of the recipes but I would like you to accept it as a gift, and an honor from a great fan of yours, and for you to add to your collections and display.

Even though I have never met you personally, I greatly admire you for being a friend and caretaker to Ron Guidry and for an incident that happened to Ron's brother, Travis, that you were a part of at a Texas Rangers' ballgame during the time of your managing the Yanks when Ron was still playing ball.

We had gone up to watch the games and while Ron's mother would always sit behind home plate, I would always purchase tickets in the first row along the third-base line, where Travis would get to see the Yankees coming onto the field from the locker room. (Travis is handicapped and does not understand the aspects of the game but does know some or most of the Yankees.)

There were many kids hanging around the area that day with the hope of getting an autograph. Some of the kids were yelling, "Yogi, Yogi." Travis would hear the kids and would ask me, "Hey Rags (that's my nickname and what Travis calls me), where's Yogi?" He was doing this both days so therefore on the last day, when Ron came over to the hotel to see us, I asked if he would ask you to come to the fence to shake hands with Travis. Ron replied that he did not know if you would do it but he would ask.

Now on that last day, all the players were on the field prior to the start of the game and I noticed Ron run up to you around second base and then both of you turned around to come toward us. Well, while you were approaching there was a crowd of fans standing in front of us, plus a big man standing in front of Travis, and there was no way for us to get to the fence. I asked him to allow Travis to go to the front because Ron and Yogi were coming to meet him. He looked at me with a sneer and frown and said, "As if."

On your and Ron's arrival, Ron could see me but not Travis and he asked, "Where is Travis?" I replied, here in front of me but this man would not allow Travis to go forward.

At that time you put out your long arms and said, "Let that boy through," and they did. Travis went forward and you spoke to him and shook his hand. Ron gave his little brother a hug and said, "I'll see you at home soon." Travis was very excited and told the kids, "Yogi just shook my hand." He was envied by all the kids present. Some even shook *his* hand.

In a sense, Rags Guidry's booklet was written like a memoir, a window into the life of a proud — and well-fed — Louisiana Cajun. Berra obviously did not have to go to Louisiana to please the Guidry family. He had done more than enough when he'd taken that walk from second base to shake Travis's hand, and that — along with his appreciation of fried frog legs and the man who prepared them for him — was apparently quite enough for Rags to title his page-two essay "A Tribute to Yogi Berra."

The Guidry men — Roland and Ron — were blessed with long memories. The seventies were ancient history, but they hadn't forgotten what Berra had done for them. Repayment would apparently entail a lifetime of kindness, along with an all-Berra-could-eat buffet.

11

Swish Hitting

Yogi Berra sat alongside Ron Guidry at the far end of the bench by the water cooler, minding his own business. In the years after Joe Torre's departure, Guidry was no longer part of the central brain trust and had moved down to the far end of the dugout. Berra followed, switching positions, just as he went from catcher to left field late in his playing career.

Joe Girardi relied much more on data than the old-school Torre, which was why general manager Brian Cashman had been an agent for change of managers and pitching coaches after the 2007 season. Berra liked Girardi very much but didn't relate to the new-age approach, and he didn't have the same history and generational comfort as with Torre.

But Berra's move away from the manager and closer to his friend Guidry also reflected the natural disengagement that inevitably comes with advanced age.

Berra, almost eighty-five, moved more slowly now. His voice was softer, harder to project. It was spring training 2010, and he understandably had become more reticent about volunteering hitting or fielding tips, not wanting to impose himself on the players when he had something to say. Instead, he told Guidry.

On this pleasant night at George M. Steinbrenner Field, they were watching Nick Swisher bat against a right-handed pitcher whose name was not especially memorable in the blur of meaningless exhibitions.

The man they called "Swish" was a cross between your friendly neighborhood bartender and the prototypical "clown prince," the life of a generally staid clubhouse in serious need of levity since the team had moved across the street into its spacious and luxurious new digs in 2009. But now Swisher was in a spring training slump that had him kicking dirt and flinging his helmet after the pitcher threw a sinkerball that he swung over for a harmless roller to second base.

As it happened, Berra recalled the previous night's game, when Swisher had produced the same result against another breaking-ball pitcher. "You know," Berra said, leaning in to Guidry, "he just needs to move up in the box. This guy's not throwing hard enough to bust it by him."

Guidry nodded. That made sense. If Swisher was standing too far back, the ball would dip under his swing, and the best he could do was hit it weakly on the ground.

"Shit," Guidry said, "why don't you tell that to *him?*"

Berra shook his head. "Nah," he said. "I don't like doing that. He's already got a hitting coach."

Guidry knew darn well that no Yankee in his right mind — much less one worth his pinstripes — would have the nerve not to welcome the advice of Yogi Berra. But he also knew what Berra was thinking and probably getting at: he was too old now for players to take seriously.

Guidry hated the sound of surrender from this man whose opinion and expertise had meant so much. For sure, Berra still loved bantering with the players, showing up first thing every morning, waiting for them to arrive so he could make the rounds. The career, or core, Yankees — Mariano Rivera, Jorge Posada, Andy Pettitte, and Derek Jeter — found Berra to be a particularly welcoming sight.

"I think that's what makes our organization special, and it's not taking anything away from anyone else, any other organization, but we have an opportunity to mingle with someone like Yogi," Jeter said. Yes, he realized, the Red Sox had their own organizational Yogi in Johnny Pesky—for whom the right-field foul pole at Fenway Park was named—and the Cardinals had Red Schoendienst in their camp over the years. But in Jeter's mind, Berra was the brand name of inspirational elders—not that there was much Berra could have taught Jeter at this point in his career.

Like Berra, Jeter was a master at not overthinking the game, keeping it simple, doing what came naturally, without letting anyone—most of all the media—distract him. Few, in fact, were allowed past the invisible moat Jeter constructed around himself, Berra being one of the exceptions. "He's special, someone who keeps the tradition and the mystique alive," Jeter said. "Me and Yogi have always had a good relationship. We tease each other."

By spring training 2010, Berra's newest dig at Jeter was that his fifth championship ring, secured in the 2009 World Series, placed him exactly halfway to Berra's total of ten.

"Yeah," Jeter would say, "but there were no playoffs when you played, so in reality we're tied."

Berra would wave a hand and say, "If you don't win the series, it don't count."

These were the baseball moments Berra lived for, his face lighting up when one of the players took the time to kibitz with him. He was grateful for the attention, but sometimes it grated on Guidry. He was convinced that Berra still had more important things to offer. He especially didn't appreciate the idea of Berra being reduced to the level of mascot—however beloved—and took it upon himself to watch out for anyone having too much fun at Berra's expense.

When the young pitcher Joba Chamberlain was pulled over and cited for drunk driving by Nebraska police in 2008, he tried to schmooze the officer with inside baseball talk. When he mentioned knowing the great Yogi Berra, he cracked, "He might not be as tall as the front of your car." Chamberlain was embarrassed when his remark went viral on the Internet after surfacing in a police video. Knowing it sounded disrespectful, he called Berra to apologize.

Ray Negron — the longtime Steinbrenner protégé who had been around since the seventies — once in a while stretched the limits of teasing with Berra, whom he had long ago taken to calling Larry. Guidry didn't like the tone of the dialogue one day and threatened to deposit the middle-aged but still playful Negron in the wastebasket — as Sparky Lyle had done three decades ago when Negron had gotten on his nerves.

It ate at Guidry that anyone, and most of all the younger Yankees, might not show Berra the proper respect. They needed to know everything the man represented, all that he still had stored in that steel trap of a baseball mind. As he sat on the bench after Swisher's groundout, Guidry asked himself, "Why shouldn't Berra share his opinion? What the hell did age have to do with it?"

"Yogi was a guy who had already been through the same damn thing, and a lot longer than any of the coaches," he said.

When Swisher returned to the dugout, ambled down the steps and past the bat rack, and, almost on cue, proceeded to march down the row in the direction of the water cooler, Guidry stood up suddenly and blocked his path. He pointed an index finger at Berra.

"He wants to talk to you," he said.

Swisher was momentarily startled but obediently sat down in the space Guidry had vacated. No stranger to Berra, or anyone else around the clubhouse, Swisher, for one, didn't think Berra needed much defending, though he understood and marveled at how Guidry looked out for him.

"There's that difference of making sure that man's respected and not put in a spot where he gets embarrassed," said Swisher, who nonetheless refused to sell Berra short in a friendly war of wits. "I'm telling you, it's crazy, but Yogi's a good counterpuncher. You can come with a quick jab, but he'll come right back over the top with something."

Swisher believed this was the blessing of ongoing engagement, the fierce determination of Berra to remain connected to his favorite pastimes — baseball and the Yankees — long after people his age or even younger tend to stop fine-tuning their bodies and minds.

"I think some of that comes from just being in this locker room, man, because when you come in here, you had better be quick-witted with all the trash-talking going on," Swisher said. "Yogi's not scared to bust people now and then. It shocks me sometimes how sharp his mind is."

The clubhouse in the new Yankee Stadium — in which every player's personal space came fully computer loaded — was more full-service hotel than fraternal jock hostel. Berra, for one, missed the intimacy of the old no-frills clubhouse in the way aging newspapermen romanticized the cluttered, frenzied newsrooms that had inexorably given way to cleaner, brighter spaces devoid of atmosphere.

That may have been why Berra liked Swisher so much. If there was one area where he could count on some kind of ruckus, it was Swisher's. The switch-hitting outfielder was often entertaining someone with his high-octane personality, making everyone feel at home, even though 2009 had been Swisher's first season with the Yankees after being acquired from the White Sox.

Berra was also mindful that Swisher had catcher's roots and old-school baseball values. His father, Steve, had played the position for nine years in the midseventies to early eighties, mostly with the Cubs and Cardinals. Steve Swisher never made silly baseball money. When his playing career ended and he found work coaching in the minors, he still had to work during the off-season. His son grew up in a household in which the game was much more closely aligned with the real world.

In the Swisher home, Berra was baseball royalty, because a major-league catcher could best appreciate Berra's extraordinary body of work. Steve Swisher passed that appreciation along to his son, who had watched grainy old films of Berra and was amazed that a man his size could launch home runs in the old Yankee Stadium, where the fences were significantly deeper in the gaps and to dead center than those in the new stadium.

"Yogi, man, your bat was always moving," Swisher told him. Berra explained that his bat was so heavy, he needed to stay flexible to generate a quick swing.

When Swisher checked Berra's career batting statistics — .285 average, 358 home runs (eleven seasons with 20 or more), and 1,430 runs batted in (with a single-season high of 125) — he was even more impressed.

"From having grown up with my dad, I always knew that being an everyday catcher is a grimy job — one hundred fifty/one hundred fifty-five games a season," Swisher said. "Just to be able to do that, be solid defensively, a standup guy, a leader, and a respected teammate, that's a major thing for me, man. Yogi did all that, and then he won three MVPs, which I'm not sure many people even know or remember. And on top of that, you got the ten rings, which he always lets you know about."

Attempting his own Yogi imitation, Swisher said, "He comes up to me after we won the series in '09 and says, 'Congratulations, you're only nine behind me.' I cracked up, man. I told him, 'Yogi, you remind me so much of my grandfather.'" Swisher lived with his paternal grandparents after his parents divorced when he was eleven. Don Swisher was a career-long security guard for DuPont back home in Parkersburg, West Virginia, known around town as "Hot Donny." He died in 2008, three years after his wife, Betty. After getting to know Berra in New York, Swisher told him that he was adopting Berra as his surrogate grandfather.

"The thing is that baseball is a lot different nowadays," Swisher said. "These days, twenty minutes after the game, everybody's out of the clubhouse. I remember my dad telling me stories, man, guys sitting around for two hours afterward, talking about the game, this and that, and that's what I like about guys like Yogi and Gator. They want to be around, talking about the game, all the little things. So when

Gator told me that Yogi wanted to talk to me, it was, like, hell, yes. I automatically figured he had something he must have seen."

Swisher sat down and put his arm on Berra's shoulder. "Yogi, these guys are wearing me out, man," he said.

The grand elder who had heard it all before, Berra leaned forward and into Swisher so that their shoulders were touching. He was aware that his voice no longer projected, and in the clatter of the dugout, he wanted to make sure that Swisher could hear him. Swisher moved his face close to Berra's and put his arm around Yogi's shoulders.

"Listen," Berra said, "all you need to do is take a step toward the plate and a step toward the pitcher. You're letting the pitch break down on you too much. That's why these guys are getting you out. Don't worry about the fastball. He can't get it by you. His best pitch is going down and away."

Swisher listened carefully, nodding again and again.

"That's it?" he said.

"That's it," Berra said.

"Yogi, man, I appreciate that," Swisher said. "I really do."

He promised to take the advice and to move up in the box in his next at bat. When his turn in the order came around again, with the same pitcher still on the mound, Swisher got into his swing early and powered the ball into the opposite-field gap, up against the wall for a standup double. Standing on second base with a shit-eating grin, he looked into the dugout, trying to make eye contact with Berra, who was already watching the next hitter dig in, oblivious to Swisher. Guidry had to grab his arm and say, "Hey, he's trying to tell you something."

When Berra turned his attention back to second, Swisher was pointing both fingers at him. Scoring a couple of minutes later, Swisher rolled back into the dugout and squeezed onto the bench alongside Berra, who was beaming, feeling like a coach all over again.

"You see?" he said. "All you have to do is make contact with the baseball, move up against a breaking-ball pitcher, step into it from your back side."

"You mean that's all you tried to do, two little keys?" Swisher said. Berra shrugged. *That's all it was.*

Swisher had to admit that he tended at times to analyze "every little thing in the swing rather than just doing what you have to do, and that's make contact with the baseball."

"Yeah, I was a pretty simple hitter," Berra said. "All this breaking down the swing stuff — never did none of that."

As it turned out, in 2010 Swisher went on to post career highs in hits (163), batting average (.288), and slugging percentage (.511) while hitting 29 home runs and driving in 89. He insisted that Berra's tip helped, especially during slumps, although Guidry said that in the grand scheme of things, whether it helped or not didn't really matter.

"Whether Yogi had anything to do with the season Swisher had — who knows?" he said. "That's immaterial." All Guidry knew while watching the episode unfold — from Berra's first comment to the look on his face when Swisher returned to the dugout to continue the conversation — was that Guidry was left with a triumphant sense of mission accomplished.

"From Swisher's point of view, he sat down and talked to Yogi and then went right up there and hit the ball to the damn wall," Guidry said. "That's what made the moment so special — something immediate came out of it. And that's all that really mattered — Swisher accepted what Yogi told him, and the way it turned out, he didn't waste his time. And in Yogi's mind, he felt, *OK, it justifies me being here.* Everybody loves having him anyway, but I know for a fact that he's not thinking that. What he's thinking is that he was still able to contribute something."

With an assist from Guidry, that is, and with classic Berra brevity, he acknowledged as much when he was asked about the session with Swisher. "Gator made me," he said.

Months later, Guidry sat in the dugout at Yankee Stadium, catching up with his pal Goose Gossage on Old-Timers' Day, an occasion they enthusiastically looked forward to every season, taking pride in its enduring tradition.

"I mean, if you take Old-Timers' Day out of the picture, if you don't celebrate the past and these great relationships and what the game stands for, why the hell are we all here in the first place?" Guidry said. "It's about what it means to wear a Yankees cap, a uniform, and the fact is that we still have it. We're the only ones, and you have to ask yourself, 'Why is that? Why not the Dodgers? They're a great franchise. Why not Boston? They've got a lot of great old-timers. Why do we keep this tradition and no one else does?'"

Calling Old-Timers' Day his "favorite day of the year," Swisher said that as a relative newcomer and someone who had experienced major-league baseball on the West Coast (Oakland) and in the Midwest (Chicago), the answer was obvious. "That breaks down from the top," he said. "There's nothing else in baseball like that, and that started with George Steinbrenner."

Although Steinbrenner had indisputably restored the Yankees' sense of manifest destiny, the truth is that the tradition of Old-Timers' Day predated Steinbrenner by decades, the first official one being staged in 1946. And while he continued it after all the imitators gave up, the event remained subject to the Boss's competitive and occasionally imperious quirks.

One regrettable change he made was abandoning the long-standing routine of having the former players dress in the clubhouse, assigning one old-timer to each active dressing stall to share with a current player. "Let me tell you, there was nothing better as an active player than to sit in the clubhouse and watch those guys—Mickey and Whitey and the rest of them—come in and start telling their stories," Gossage said.

Whoever was assigned to his space—Gossage recalled hosting the old right-hander Ralph Terry from the great early-sixties teams at least twice—he would say, "Hey, it's all yours today." All Gossage wanted was to be a fly on the wall, soak it all in. But when the Yankees blew a game one Old-Timers' Day, Steinbrenner decided the crowd in the clubhouse had been a distraction and had the old-timers moved into their own room the following year.

That left the dugout as the best place for the generations to meet and mingle. But in 2010, when Guidry and Gossage looked around during the annual reenactment of two or three innings, they were startled by how few active players had left the comfort of the clubhouse to fraternize with the old-timers.

"I was like, 'Where the hell are these guys?'" Gossage said. "When we played, we'd all be out there. It was expected, but no one had to actually tell you or ask. You wanted to be out there. To be honest, I was kind of shocked."

He wondered if all the comings and goings of modern baseball, the revolving-door rosters, were taking their toll even on the Yankees. Guidry had considered that possibility himself. But at least Swisher was out there, clowning with everyone, along with the core four — Jeter, Posada, Pettitte, and the incomparable Mo Rivera.

"Gator, I want to see what you got left," Rivera said.

Guidry laughed, and Gossage butted in to defend Guidry's — and his own — honor by insisting that Guidry had enough to get through one lousy inning — which was all the modern-day closer needed to work in any given game to become an all-time legend.

The first time Guidry laid eyes on Mariano Rivera, he thought he was looking at a Latino version of his younger self. It was 1993, on a back field of the Yankees' old spring training complex in Fort Lauderdale, the area reserved for fresh-faced kids trying to climb their way up the minor-league ladder.

"We used to call it Iwo Jima, because when we first started out, it was just an infield with sand in the back of it," Guidry said, meaning there was no outfield grass. "When we practiced, we actually used to have to watch out for snakes."

The complex had been upgraded and landscaped by the time Rivera signed with the Yankees for $3,000 as an undrafted player out of Panama City in 1990. The son of a fishing boat captain, Rivera spoke no English and had never heard of Ron Guidry, much less Yogi Berra.

"I played baseball, but I didn't know anything about the game in America," he said. "I knew about soccer. Even when I was already two/three years in the organization, I didn't know anything. I knew the game. I saw the players and all that stuff, on TV. But that was it."

The year Rivera showed up on Guidry's radar, he was mostly concerned with preserving a career, rehabbing from surgery in August 1992 to repair damage to the ulnar collateral ligament in his right elbow. That November, he was left unprotected by the Yankees in the draft to stock the two new expansion teams, the Florida Marlins and Colorado Rockies. Both passed on him. When Rivera reported to Fort Lauderdale the following spring, Guidry was asked to take a look at the young right-hander, who was coming off elbow surgery.

Guidry went to the back fields, asked around for Rivera, settled behind the batting cage to watch him throw, and fell in love at first sight. Here was this rail-thin minor-leaguer with a relaxed, easy motion and a fastball that exploded into the catcher's glove, belying the near-hypnotic fluidity of his delivery.

"You could see the pop and the movement, and I'm saying, 'How long ago was the surgery, less than a year?'" Guidry said. "Then I find out he's not that young, already twenty-three, and I say, 'Hmm, I think I've heard this story before.'"

When Rivera was finished throwing, Guidry introduced himself, and they sat on a tarp by the side of the field. He had been told that Rivera's English wasn't good, but there was something about the way he listened, his earnest expression, that made Guidry believe that communication was not going to be much of a problem.

"OK, you just had an injury, you're not going to be doing very much this year, so make sure you take time to heal it," Guidry told him. "Just do a little easy throwing, nothing strenuous. Please don't let them talk you into hurrying up and trying to come back. You got a great arm; you're probably not going anywhere."

Nobody knew better than Guidry that certainty did not exist for a young pitcher in the organization, not in those pre-championship days and with Steinbrenner agitating for instant gratification. But Guidry sensed that the Yankees might have something special in this deeply religious man. He hoped they would keep the faith.

"There are guys that you can just watch and know that they're going to be special if given the opportunity," he said. "And Mo with a baseball in his hand was like Rembrandt with a paintbrush."

When he noticed Steinbrenner lurking in the area one day while Rivera was throwing batting practice, Guidry offered his two cents, reminding the Boss of how impatient he had been with another young flamethrower and late bloomer.

"Mr. Steinbrenner," he said, "when you start making trades, do not include this kid. If you lose him, you'll never win."

Steinbrenner nodded, thanked Guidry for the insight, and two years later tried to trade Rivera and Jorge Posada to the Cincinnati Reds for David Wells. Fortunately for him, the offer was refused. In 1997, Rivera inherited the closer's role from John Wetteland. He then became the greatest closer that baseball has ever known.

There was no other contemporary Yankee that Guidry was closer to than Rivera, no player he respected and appreciated more. He related to Rivera's minimalist nature, how he had become one of the most understated superstars in the history of American team sports, a power pitcher who intimidated without threatening hitters or showing them up.

His mesmerizing aura was based purely on performance in an era of wanton — and often rewarding — pomposity. When Rivera dispensed criticism or support for teammates, they always listened, because his words were never used frivolously. When he became the star of an advertising campaign for Canali, a high-end Italian clothing company, he did not suffer the fraternal clubhouse abuse he predicted he would. Even Swisher, the leading candidate for comic antagonist, gave him a pass.

Deeply religious and family oriented, Rivera was popular with younger teammates and retired legends alike. They all respected his space, the way he carried himself and wore his pinstripes.

"Mo is very special to me," Guidry said. "I mean, he reminded me so much of myself when I first saw him."

It wasn't just his velocity in relation to his physique, or that he was in his midtwenties when he reached the majors, or that Steinbrenner had tried to get rid of him. It was the way he conditioned himself, how beautifully he fielded his position, how much he made pitching synonymous with athleticism, as had Guidry.

"I remember him in his twenties, when everyone else was twenty yards behind him when he was running," Guidry said. Eighteen years Rivera's senior, Guidry would tease him, "One of these days, you're going to be just like I am—old." And while in 2010 Rivera was still an extraordinarily dominant closer beyond age forty, Guidry watched him closely in spring training. He was taking it easier, shaking his head as the young kids blew by him. "You told me this would happen," Rivera told Guidry. "Yeah, I remember."

Back home in Louisiana, on the couch in front of his flat-screen TV, Guidry watched a grounder scoot under Rivera's glove one day, a play he would once have made effortlessly. Guidry dialed Steve Donohue's cell phone and left a message for the assistant trainer. "Tell Mo I'm calling every time that happens from now on," he said. "Tell him that's what happens when you get old."

Guidry knew that Rivera would take it the right way, laughing it off for the good-natured gibe that it was. More than teammates, Guidry and Rivera were members of a grand social order. The core Yankees—Rivera, Jeter, Pettitte, and Posada—all belonged to that order, as did Bernie Williams, who adored Berra, along with others from the nineties nucleus. They marveled and were moved by the Berra-Guidry relationship and recognized the reciprocal nature of the generational bonding.

"I'm pretty sure there was a time when Yogi took care of Gator, you know what I mean?" Jeter said, guessing correctly.

When Brian Cashman, the longtime general manager who started as a front office intern in 1986, was asked which of the contemporary players reminded him most of Guidry and Berra, he cited one player, unhesitatingly. "In our clubhouse, the one guy who is most like them is Mo, because he sees the game the same way, as a family structure," Cashman said. "Those guys are rare, far from the norm. They believe that taking care of one another and treating people the right way no matter how much success they've had is part of the job."

The more bats he broke with his classic split-fingered fastball, the more Rivera caught up on his Yankees history. He watched the videos, filled in the blanks of his Central American childhood. He became a regular stop on Berra's clubhouse roaming, fascinated by the story behind Yogi's fourteen-year absence and reemergence. Unless he was pressed, Rivera didn't say a whole lot, but there was little he didn't see.

He took special note of the relationship between Berra and Guidry, watching them come and go over the years. "That is real love, something very special," he said.

From their first conversation on the back fields of Fort Lauderdale, Rivera's friendship with Guidry also evolved as a subtext to Guidry and Berra's relationship. Early every spring, when pitchers strengthen their arms with long tossing drills, Rivera typically chose Guidry as his partner, even as Guidry pushed sixty and his stamina began to fade. "I wouldn't tell that son of a gun that I had to ice my arm every day," Guidry said, stubborn to the point of pain.

On the average day, he was good for about twenty long tosses right into Rivera's chest before fatigue would set in. But Guidry's throws lost steam, and fewer went where he wanted them to go. "So what would Mo do?" Guidry said. "He'd take a couple of steps forward to make it easier for me."

Just as Guidry took care of Berra on the golf course, Rivera made sure Guidry was not embarrassed on the ball field. He did it without having to be asked, because as Guidry said, "There are unspoken things, part of the camaraderie and trust."

And while Guidry wasn't planning to be around spring training when he was eighty, he could imagine himself back at Yankee Stadium on some future Old-Timers' Day, old and rickety, but still spry enough to climb the dugout steps and wave his cap once more to the crowd.

Which younger Yankees legend would be perfectly positioned to watch out for him as he planted a foot on that first step? Who would remind him to go slow, as Guidry had done for Berra, standing guard in the years after his return? He couldn't think of any man he would rather have save him from a fall than Mariano Rivera.

Yogi had paid Nick Swisher a well-timed favor in giving the small but consequential batting tip. Now it was Swisher's turn to return it. Unfortunately, he nearly overslept.

On the morning of June 6, 2011, Swisher blinked open his eyes in the bedroom of his Manhattan high-rise apartment in a state of disorientation that comes with jet lag. Having plopped his head on the pillow about six hours earlier after a cross-country flight from Southern California, Swisher wasn't quite sure what day it was, what planet he was on, or why he was awake in the first place.

But the clock he was staring at read 9:25, and somehow that set off an alarm in his head. "Oh, shit," he said. "Yogi's gonna kick my ass!"

Swisher jumped out of bed and yelled for his wife, actress JoAnna Garcia, to come to his aid. He suddenly remembered that the limo he had arranged for would be arriving in five minutes.

"Honey," he asked his wife of six months, "can you lay out my clothes for me? I got a car coming. I can't miss Yogi's thing."

Swisher made a beeline for the shower, not even bothering to lather up.

What goes around comes around. Swisher had agreed to appear at Berra's 2011 charity golf tournament weeks earlier, despite the fact that it was on the morning after the Yankees had completed a West Coast swing with a Sunday afternoon game against the Angels in Anaheim and a long flight home.

Monday was a day off for the Yankees before the start of a series against the Red Sox at Yankee Stadium, an opportunity to sleep in, spend a lazy day in front of the television, and have a quiet dinner. But when Berra had made the rounds in the clubhouse, handing out invitations to the event as he customarily did, Swisher had promised to attend, no ifs, ands, or buts. "See, it wasn't about me, it was about him," Swisher said. "He took the time to come into the clubhouse and personally ask."

How do you say no to your appointed surrogate grandfather? In the months after Berra had told him to move up in the batter's box, Swisher had stepped up and shown Berra how much his friendship meant.

Swisher had flown his father in from West Virginia to play a round of golf and to formally introduce him to Berra at Yogi's 2010 tournament. He had invited Yogi and Carmen to his wedding in Palm Beach, Florida, in early December (the Berras couldn't attend), and months later he had asked Berra to be his presenter when he'd received an award at the annual Thurman Munson Awards Dinner in Manhattan.

There was no shortage of familiar names and faces at Berra's 2011 outing, enough to make it what Rudy Giuliani, one of the first to arrive, called "the best golf outing of the year with the best guy in sports." In his first year of retirement, Andy Pettitte flew up from Texas. Joe Torre showed up with his arm in a sling after surgery and rode around in a cart, catching up with the likes of Ralph Branca, Mike Torrez, Ron Blomberg, Rick Cerone, David Cone, Bud Harrelson, Mickey Rivers, and a few athletes from other sports who lived in the area.

Guidry, of course, blew in from Louisiana, entering with a flourish of sarcasm, demanding to know if his portly ex-teammate, Cerone the catcher, had ever been acquainted with a salad. But as much as Guidry could be the life of the party, he kept an eye out for Berra. When the call from the loudspeaker came for the golfers to descend from the breakfast terrace to the putting green, Guidry made sure he was waiting by the stairs to help Berra down. The Florida rules were in effect in New Jersey, too.

That was also about the time that Swisher burst in, apologizing to anyone who would listen for being late. Berra was so thrilled that he'd come, he didn't so much as tap his watch.

Three coaches from Joe Girardi's staff—Mick Kelleher, Larry Rothschild, and Robby Thompson—showed up while Girardi tended to another commitment. But several Yankees who had said they would try to attend did not. Only Swisher dragged himself out of bed as he promised he would. "I know it was a tough turnaround, but frankly I was surprised there weren't more guys there when, you know, it had been on the schedule for a month," he said.

At the dinner that evening, long after the day's double and triple bogeys were forgiven and forgotten, Berra was handed the microphone to say a few words to his guests. As usual, he tried to say as little as he could get away with.

"I want to especially thank the coaches and Swish," he said. "These guys, they came from the West Coast last night, almost no sleep, just to be here. They . . . they . . . what they did for us . . ."

That was it. He couldn't continue. He wiped his eyes and handed the mike to someone else. But the emotion in his voice and his glistening eyes had said it all.

12

A Yankee's Calling

Yogi Berra telephoned George Steinbrenner at his home in Tampa on the Boss's eightieth birthday. "Only a few people have the number," he said with pride, though he used it sparingly and judiciously, making sure to call Steinbrenner every Independence Day to wish him well.

On this Sunday morning, July 4, 2010, Berra thought that the ailing Steinbrenner seemed more alert than in their previous conversation, a little perkier and more playful. "How's my girlfriend?" he asked Berra, referring to Carmen.

They spoke for a couple of minutes, and Steinbrenner told him, optimistically, "Maybe I'll see you at Old-Timers' Day." That would be great, Berra said. He would look forward to it. He hung up the telephone feeling upbeat.

Berra didn't call many people on their birthdays, and he joked that the list was forever dwindling, a sad byproduct of fatal attrition. Yet even as Steinbrenner had deteriorated and virtually disappeared from public view, it never occurred to Berra that he might outlive the Boss. Even to a baseball man as iconic as Berra, Steinbrenner was an outsize personality, guaranteed to stir one's emotions, one way or another. But Berra did not derive any satisfaction from the irony that he had become a far more visible presence around the new Yankee Stadium than the man who was responsible for his fourteen-year absence from the old one. The famous feud was ancient history as far as he was concerned.

In the years following Berra's return, he and Steinbrenner had become the oddest of amicable couples. They didn't socialize but looked forward to seeing each other in spring training and at the stadium, the Boss clearly aware of the fact that Berra's presence was proof of his good heart.

And Berra, too, seemed pleased with his ability to have risen above his own resentment and rancor. When he went to a regular-season game, the first question he asked of the parking lot security guard was whether Steinbrenner was expected in the house that day. For reasons he couldn't explain, Berra got a devilish kick out of knowing the commotion there would be if the Boss was coming, along with a few fairly interesting guests.

He never knew who he might run into on his way up to Steinbrenner's box. One day, while he was waiting for the elevator, it was Michael Jordan. Berra's eyes widened, but it was Jordan who was awestruck. "Mr. B., Mr. B.," he said, grabbing Berra's hand.

Although he chose to avoid sitting near Steinbrenner when he watched a game from the owner's box, in order to steer clear of the Boss's inevitable agitation, Berra was immune from his wrath, a made man. Steinbrenner had seen to that, making it clear to his people that Berra should get whatever he wanted.

That wasn't much, compared to other dignitaries, including some who qualified as Yankees royalty. Just the same, Steinbrenner would tug on Berra's arm every now and then and say, "I have something you may want for your museum."

One day he handed over bronzed plaques of Joe DiMaggio and Mickey Mantle that had hung on the outfield fence of the old stadium before it was renovated during the midseventies. The gifts were accepted and brought across the river to New Jersey to adorn a wall of the museum. In another section of the museum, titled "Forgiving the

Boss," there is a blown-up photo of a smiling Berra and Steinbrenner on the night of their reconciliation.

There was never any getting around the fact that Steinbrenner's bluster and sometimes brutish tendencies were anathema to Berra. But he had come around to the belief that the man should ultimately be judged on results, for delivering on his vow to restore the franchise to championship prominence and beyond after buying it from CBS in 1973.

"We went through some bad times, like everyone else," Berra said. "But he was very generous, a good man. I wish I could have played for him."

Considering Steinbrenner's unceremonious firing of Berra as manager, this sounded like quite a leap to everlasting loyalty. But after all was said and done, there was no denying that Steinbrenner loved the Yankees and had honored their winning tradition, however heavy-handedly. As far as Berra was concerned, that overrode everything, including his personal indignities.

There was also no doubt how much Steinbrenner had wanted to make amends. He had spent the better part of a decade proving it. It was Steinbrenner who had persuaded Berra to accompany the Yankees to Japan for their season-opening series in 2004 — a trip even the Boss didn't make. Berra, it seemed, was part of every important team occasion in the 2000s. He was invited to press conferences introducing the latest free agent catch, led the championship parade, and stood front and center when the city broke ground for the new stadium in 2006.

He was also honorary captain for the 2008 All-Star Game in the team's last season at the old ballpark, when it finally hit home that a sobbing, sedentary Steinbrenner was a shell of his once formidable self. If that wasn't sobering enough, Berra was one of a handful of guests invited by the Boss's people to game two of the 2009 World Series, a strange and disorienting night.

To begin with, the Yankees arranged for the New York–born rap star Jay-Z to perform his hit single "Empire State of Mind," from the best-selling album *The Blueprint 3,* accompanied by Alicia Keys. The song had served as the soundtrack for Derek Jeter's at bats during the regular season and had blasted in the clubhouse during the Yankees' celebrations after winning the division and league championship series.

An avid fan, Jay-Z had worn a Yankees cap in music videos, in magazine photos, and on album covers. He had been shown on the large center-field screen at Yankee Stadium during numerous home games throughout the regular season and the playoffs. And yet, one line from the song — "Shit, I made the Yankee hat more famous than a Yankee can" — would never have passed muster with a more attentive Steinbrenner.

But the October 2009 version of the Boss was wheelchair-bound, sitting near a large round table, blankly watching the game on a flat-screen television with none of his trademark vigor. Elaine Kaufman, the owner of Elaine's, the famous Upper East Side bar and restaurant, was there. So were Steinbrenner family members and a few minority owners.

When Berra walked in, Steinbrenner looked up through eyes that had once burned with energy but were now fading embers. With a wan smile, he reached out for Berra, who bent over to give him a hug. "Yogi," he said, barely audible. "Good to see you."

"Not one of the Boss's better days," someone whispered in Berra's ear. Yogi walked away thinking it was a cruel injustice for Steinbrenner to have become such a shell of himself. He deserved to be the Boss until the end, for better or worse.

At least there was baseball to occupy his mind. Berra settled in to watch the Yankees even the series behind the pitching of A. J. Burnett and home runs by Mark Teixeira and Hideki Matsui. But he couldn't quite shake the image of Steinbrenner in the wheelchair. It was the last time the Boss was in the house that he had built and the last time Berra saw him alive.

Nine days after he called Steinbrenner to wish him happy birthday and hung up thinking he might actually see him again on Old-

Timers' Day, Berra was reading the morning papers in his Montclair home when the telephone rang. It was a Steinbrenner family aide, calling from Tampa, to say that the Boss had suffered a heart attack and been taken to the hospital.

"No . . . no, I just talked to him," Berra protested. "He sounded OK."

But he wasn't, and a while later the second call that Berra was dreading came. It was the same family aide telling him that Steinbrenner was gone, the Boss was no more. Berra went into the other room to tell Carmen. He plopped down in his chair and sat there quietly, thinking back to that wonderful night in January 1999, ignoring all that had happened before. The inevitable tears rolled down his cheeks.

Completely lost on Berra, at least for the moment, was that after all that had gone down between them — fourteen years of famously fascinating grudge holding on his part — somebody had apparently made sure that he was on the short list of people to call.

When Ron Guidry got word of the news in steamy Louisiana, he was emotionally prepared. You didn't have to be a doctor to know that the Boss's health was deteriorating. Having lost elders in his own family, including Bonnie's parents, he had suspected for a while that Steinbrenner might not have long to go.

Unlike Berra, Guidry heard of Steinbrenner's death from the television. He and Bonnie shared a moment together, a hug, then went about their business for the day. Then Guidry, who would be leaving for New York within two days, thought about how emotional the weekend up there was going to be. Upset as he was by the news, he was also a pragmatist, able to focus on the positive. He could be sad yet thankful for what had been.

In the case of Steinbrenner, he was struck by the realization that at least the Boss had lived long enough to see the new stadium open and the Yankees win another World Series, the seventh of his ownership and the franchise's twenty-seventh overall. It was a remarkable story line, really, the Boss going out on top, the way he would have scripted it in one of the press releases that his New York–based PR heavyweight Howard Rubenstein had been knocking out on his behalf in the years since he'd dropped out of sight.

Like Berra, Guidry had long made his peace with Steinbrenner, appreciative of the fact that the volatile man who was capable of egregious mistakes was also capable of not only admitting them but making up for them as well.

Case in point: In 1978, Guidry's 25–3 season for the ages, he was named Athlete of the Year by the Associated Press. The awards dinner just happened to be in Tampa. Steinbrenner attended the banquet and asked to say a few words about his star left-hander.

He didn't beg Guidry's forgiveness, as he would with Berra twenty-one years later. But in this very public setting, he went out of his way to set the record straight.

"I almost made a big mistake in 1976 by trading this young man," he said. "I'm so glad I was talked out of it, because, as it turns out, we would never have accomplished what we did in the last couple of years if it wasn't for him."

The fact that Steinbrenner told this to the audience as opposed to saying it in private meant everything to a proud man like Guidry. Love him or hate him, he had the ability to tell the world, in effect, *I was a fool.*

"Like with Yogi, the biggest thing was that he flew from Tampa to New Jersey to apologize," Guidry said. "He didn't send a car and a plane and bring him to Tampa. He got on the damn plane himself. And if he had walked in that door and said, 'Hey, Yogi, how're you doing?' Yogi would have gone to the ballpark the next day. He wouldn't have had to say anything. But he did, because he knew it was the right thing to do. So regardless of how you felt about him as a player or as a coach — and it never was easy — you wind up realizing that he only was demanding the best and he wasn't afraid to do that, to put himself out there and not give a damn what anyone thought."

In the end, Steinbrenner had won Guidry over, convinced him

that he was much more than a rich man with some deep psychological need to control and belittle other men — what Guidry had originally believed. Knowing how it all turned out, Guidry could even smile now at the memories of Steinbrenner barging into the clubhouse, pointing fingers, making the winning and losing of a ballgame out to be life-and-death.

When one of the young Yankees would casually remark how much he would have enjoyed playing for Steinbrenner in his autocratic prime, Guidry would smirk and say, "You have no idea." It was impossible to know how anyone would react to such ribald harassment in the heat of a pennant race or an ego-deflating slump.

"He would start in — 'You and you and you!' — and then he'd tell you that he's got this multimillion-dollar business, the New York Yankees, and we're supposed to be playing like New York Yankees," Guidry said. "So he's chewing your ass out, and if you put your tail between your legs and go hide, do you know what that looks like in his eyes? It looks like he doesn't have anything.

"But if he points his finger at you and you flip him off or you tell him exactly where he can go, he's going to rant and rave and then walk outside that door and say, 'Man, I've got somebody.' He won't tell you that to your face. But deep down inside, he knows it."

Steinbrenner, Guidry said, relished the role of the imperious patriarch, never minded being the bad guy. He cited the famous *Sports Illustrated* cover of the Boss on a horse in a Napoleon outfit.

"Was Napoleon a good guy or a horrible guy?" Guidry said. "Trust me, George preferred it that way, but he actually had a heart of gold. That should be on his gravestone — no matter how he appeared on the outside, he was good on the inside."

Sitting next to her husband, Bonnie Guidry nodded, contemplating her own brushes with the Boss back in the day, or especially during her Ronnie's best days, in 1978.

On the final scheduled day of that regular season, the Yankees had come all the way back from a fourteen-game deficit to lead the Red Sox by one game with one to play. All they had to do was beat

Cleveland, a team with ninety losses, to clinch the American League East. Instead, Catfish Hunter lasted only an inning and two-thirds; the Yankees got rocked 9–2 and fell into a tie with the victorious Sox, forcing the one-game playoff at Fenway Park the next afternoon.

After the Cleveland loss, some of the Yankees' wives got together and decided that while they didn't ordinarily travel with the team, they had a right to be at Fenway the next day for what promised to be a historic game. Getting on the plane with their husbands was out of the question, but someone raised the possibility of asking the Yankees to charter a plane for them.

The outspoken Bonnie was asked to present the request to Steinbrenner. Before she had a chance to think too much about marching into the Boss's office after such a defeat — and to Cleveland, his native city, no less — she agreed. But just to be on the safe side, she asked Stormy Dent, Bucky's wife at the time, to accompany her.

Steinbrenner was in his office with the door closed when the two women presented themselves to his secretary — Doris, as Bonnie recalled — and asked if they could have a moment with the big man. Doris told them to have a seat; she would check in a couple of minutes.

Just as they sat down, the telephone rang, and the door to Steinbrenner's office opened.

"World champion New York Yankees," Doris said, answering the phone.

Appearing in the doorway, Steinbrenner furiously blurted out, "World champions? They're not *world champions*. They're chumps! World *chumps,* the way they played today!"

Bonnie looked at Stormy, thinking maybe this wasn't a good time to bring up the charter. Too late: Steinbrenner had spotted them. They didn't even get a chance to introduce themselves before he demanded, "And what do you two want?"

He took a second look and pointed to Stormy Dent. "And you, your husband, he hasn't had a damn hit in a week!"

Steinbrenner was exaggerating only slightly. Bucky Dent had gone hitless in the Cleveland series and was one for his last thirteen.

Bonnie was thankful — pleasantly surprised even — that the owner seemed to place them with their husbands. She guessed that Steinbrenner at least knew *of* her because Ron had gone in one day at her urging to demand a telephone for the players' family lounge. "Either you spend five minutes talking to me or you can talk to my wife for an hour," Guidry had said.

They got the phone. What the hell, Bonnie reasoned now; she might as well go for the plane.

"Mr. Steinbrenner, we think we should be in Boston tomorrow," she said. "We're not asking to go with the team, but we think the Yankees should get a plane for the wives."

Steinbrenner ranted some more about the Yankees losing to Cleveland and having to go to Boston at all. But later that evening, the wives boarded a charter and joined their husbands in their Boston hotel.

When Dent heard about Steinbrenner's rant from his wife, he wasn't too pleased. As fate would have it, on the Dents' way out of the hotel for a bite to eat, the elevator door opened, and there was Steinbrenner, who apparently hadn't forgotten what he'd said. He also intuitively knew it was time to make nice. "Your time will come," he told his stone-faced shortstop.

The next day, they all watched Dent crack the biggest hit of his life — a three-run homer in the seventh inning off Mike Torrez — to ignite the pennant-clinching victory.

Was it a coincidence or another instance where Steinbrenner incited a Yankee to do something heroic? Depends what kind of spin you want to put on it.

Before the playoff game, when Steinbrenner came into the clubhouse to fire up his troops, he especially wanted to have an audience with Guidry, his starting pitcher. Starting pitchers seldom want to talk to anyone before a game, and the last person Guidry wanted a pep talk from before this game was Steinbrenner. He hid under a table that was draped with a towel by the trainer, Gene Monahan. When the Boss asked where the heck Guidry was, he was told out in the bullpen, probably. Steinbrenner never found Guidry, who nonetheless appreciated the thought.

Guidry prepared rabbit stew one last time for Steinbrenner during spring training 2010. He just didn't know when he would get the opportunity to serve it, because Steinbrenner had pretty much stopped coming to the ballpark.

But when Guidry went to the annual Boys & Girls Clubs fundraising luncheon the Yankees hold every spring, lo and behold, there Steinbrenner was, in his wheelchair, sounding weak but alert enough to badger Guidry one last time.

"When are you bringing the stew?" he asked.

"You're never there," Guidry said.

"I'll be there tomorrow night," Steinbrenner said.

Guidry delivered the stew the next night and thought about the time Steinbrenner had wandered over at Grambling, where his father had done the cooking. He choked up a bit on his way down to the field, thinking about how precious time was, how important it was to not waste it. He thought about Steinbrenner and Berra and all the traditions that went with being part of the Yankees extended family.

Some traditions, he decided, are worth carrying on, no matter who is left to participate. The following year, the Yankees' first spring training without George Steinbrenner in thirty-eight years, Guidry made another rabbit stew at his apartment, brought a bowl to the ballpark the next day, and headed straight for the executive office.

There he found Jennifer Steinbrenner Swindal, a Yankees general partner and vice chairperson. "Jenny, I used to make this for your dad," he said. "I'd feel funny if I didn't offer you some."

The Boss's daughter was taken aback. Rabbit stew wasn't exactly her choice cuisine. But she was so touched by Guidry's sincerity that she took the bowl and later sat down to eat. "It was delicious," she said. "The Cajun spices were amazing."

She later tracked down Guidry, told him she loved the stew, and asked if he would continue to make it for her for as long as he came to spring training. Her father would have liked that.

On the day Steinbrenner died, the phones didn't stop ringing at the Yogi Berra Museum & Learning Center. The interview requests were countless, for obvious reasons. If anyone could speak to the paradoxical nature of the owner's personality, it was Berra, who had experienced Steinbrenner at his worst and at his absolute best.

"It was huge, oh my gosh," Jessica Steinbrenner, the Boss's other daughter, said, when asked how significant the apology to Berra was in her father's life. The gesture, she said, was probably the most vulnerable the Boss had ever allowed himself to be as an adult.

"There were times that Dad had been overwhelmed by emotion and reduced to tears, but making up with Yogi may have been the biggest, most emotional, and best thing he'd ever done," she said. "For all his temper and lashing out, he was able to be reflective and come to a middle ground to remedy a terrible mistake."

It wasn't long after Steinbrenner's apology to Berra that he began to show symptoms of physical decline — unable to keep from crying in public during emotional moments, fainting in December 2003 at a funeral service for football legend Otto Graham in Florida, and moving noticeably more stiffly and slowly.

The argument could be made that Steinbrenner had acted in the nick of time with Berra, before the window closed. He wrote one of the great story lines in Yankees history and created a narrative that may have benefited no one more than himself.

"Think about how much that helped the way George was perceived as he got older," said Rick Cerrone, the former media relations director, who was with Steinbrenner that night in January 1999. "Not only was Yogi around the Yankees — which in itself was a blessing — but it put a softer face on George. It helped people really see that there was a whole different side."

This was the side that Berra chose to remember when he met with reporters in the lobby of his museum hours after learning of Steinbrenner's death. He wore a white short-sleeved shirt and a Yankees cap and was accompanied by his son Dale. Also present was Carmen, who chimed in that Steinbrenner would surprise people with acts of kindness — little things, like sending vendors to the section where the wives of players and coaches were sitting to bring them cotton candy during a World Series game.

Berra pointed out that while people criticized Steinbrenner for buying the best free agents with enhanced Yankees revenue streams, he was the one who had created those streams. People had to admit that Steinbrenner was only playing by baseball's modern rules and that he had adapted to them better than anyone else.

Berra didn't want to sound as though he was blind to Steinbrenner's imperfections. For one thing, Berra wished that the Boss could have settled all his old scores. It bothered him that Joe Torre and Don Zimmer, in particular, had had messy divorces with Steinbrenner and the Yankees and would never get the chance to reconcile with the Boss.

He could smile at the memory of how upset Steinbrenner had been on the October night in 1999 when Zimmer was struck in the face by a foul ball. Berra and the Boss had hustled from his box into the elevator and down to the clubhouse, where Zimmer thought he was seeing things when the cobwebs cleared and he saw their concerned faces hovering over him.

Zimmer's habit of speaking his mind, of not tolerating Steinbrenner's antics, ultimately got him on the Boss's bad side and led to his angry exit from the franchise in 2003. Zimmer further antagonized Steinbrenner in a tell-all book two years later.

Torre's situation was much different. Although he had his share of run-ins with Steinbrenner over his twelve years as manager, most of them were kept private — at least until the end of his tenure, in 2007, when the Yankees staged a public and tortured contract negotiation that led to his resignation. Torre knew there were others in the organization hankering for change and, more important, that the Boss was not well. Just the same, he later asked Berra, "How long did you stay away?"

"Me? Fourteen years."

"I might be gone longer than that," Torre said, admitting that the publication of his book, *The Yankee Years,* in 2009 had infuriated many in the organization and wasn't about to land him on the guest list anytime soon.

But by the fall of 2010, there was no point in either party perpetuating a feud that seemed unnecessarily petty in the aftermath of Steinbrenner's death. Torre returned to the Bronx and stepped into the new stadium for the first time that September when the Yankees unveiled a monument to their fallen owner.

No one could argue that the Boss didn't deserve one, but everyone, Berra included, was struck by its size. It loomed over the ballpark like the visage of a Third-World dictator. Berra shrugged when someone noted that it was double the size of Babe Ruth's and laughed when another Yankees insider joked that it was probably visible from outer space.

But Berra would not personally engage in any Steinbrenner bashing, not a single word, and he wouldn't take kindly to anyone else's criticism that at least wasn't laced with humor. That was something Guidry had noticed in the years since Berra had returned to the Yankees. "You can't say anything bad about George around Yogi," Guidry said. "If you do, he'll give you a look. That's just the way it is, just where Yogi was."

Berra was back inside the Steinbrenner circle and hoping to land in the winner's circle after Jessica Steinbrenner, who handled the family's thoroughbred operation in Ocala, Florida, named a promising colt Yogi Berra — just as she had named one Boss Yankee for her father.

When she asked Berra's permission, he was flattered. "Sure," he said. But a few months later, when he ran into Jessica in the family box, Berra, not exactly enlightened on the developmental timeline of a thoroughbred, wanted to know if his namesake had won anything yet.

"Yogi, we have to wait two years before we run him," she said.

He frowned and shook his head. "I hope I'm alive in two years," he said, perhaps thinking of Jessica's father.

She squeezed his arm, flashed a warm smile, and said, "Something to look forward to."

13

Concessions

Something weighed heavily on Yogi Berra as he arrived at spring training 2011. It was a subject he had broached with Carmen at home and Dave Kaplan at the museum before leaving New Jersey but now had to run past Ron Guidry, whose opinion would matter most.

Mindful of the toll that his fall of the previous summer had taken and worried that he could no longer deal with the rigors of daily participation in the spring training routine, Berra posed the question to Guidry in the form of a childlike plea: "It's OK I don't wear the uniform, isn't it?"

The question surprised Guidry—though not because he hadn't considered the possibility that Berra might not be spry enough to clomp around in cleats and a baseball suit anymore. It was more the innocence of the phrasing, the notion that Berra might actually need permission and that someone might disapprove of him hanging around the clubhouse without the familiar number 8 on his back.

But Guidry soon came around to the realization that Berra wasn't really asking as much as he was coming to grips with the uneasy transition in his own mind. Guidry had once been forced to pull off the road in a fit of convulsive laughter when Berra had told him he had to shoot an "affliction commercial." Now Guidry seized up, grit his teeth, and gripped the wheel tightly. How difficult, he thought, it must have been for Berra to reach the conclusion that he could no longer dress the part of the forever Yankee, as he had for more than six decades — excluding his self-imposed exile, when his baseball wardrobe had been limited to the cap.

The cap he had never stopped wearing.

"It's OK, Yogi," Guidry said, nodding. "No one's going to mind."

And one more thing, Berra said. He wouldn't be in the dugout with Guidry anymore for the exhibition games. Even if that were allowed, under no circumstances would he let himself be down there dressed as a civilian.

"You don't need to be sitting in no dugout," Guidry told him. "Go upstairs where it's comfortable, it's air-conditioned, where they got food."

The next day, Berra still insisted on arriving just after the birds began chirping. Wearing a blue Yankees windbreaker and cap, he made his way into Joe Girardi's office before catching up with the regulars — trainers Gene Monahan and Steve Donohue, old hands Derek Jeter and Mariano Rivera, and of course his pal Nick Swisher.

He also made sure to shake hands with the new starting catcher, Russell Martin, who remembered the time he looked up from his dressing stall in the Dodgers' clubhouse at Shea Stadium and did a double take as Berra strolled by. "Holy shit," he said to himself. "That's Yogi Bleeping Berra."

On the afternoon of the first game, Berra took the elevator upstairs to one of the executive suites. He was accompanied by Lou Cucuzza Jr., whose father, Lou Cucuzza Sr., had preceded him as the clubhouse manager and many days could be heard bellowing in the corridor of Yankee Stadium, "Make way, Hall of Famer coming through," as he transported Berra from one clubhouse to another by cart.

Before going up, Berra told Guidry that he didn't think he would want to stay for the whole game — another concession, damn it. "Fine, you don't have to," Guidry said, thinking fast. "I'll take you back early."

Guidry asked Cucuzza to go back upstairs during the sixth inning and walk Berra back down to the clubhouse. Guidry would be waiting there for him. He would take a quick shower, get dressed, and pick up Berra's bag, then off they would go, Berra to the hotel and Guidry to his apartment, until it was time for dinner.

This quickly became the new normal, and Guidry couldn't help but feel some sadness. The fact of the matter was that he still hadn't quite adjusted to Berra's inability to play golf beyond the few ceremonial tee shots at his own tournament.

"That was hard for me, not being able to play with Yogi anymore," he said. "We always had such a good time, so much fun, with the General. It didn't feel the same without him."

Now it was Berra's proximity to the game and the many hours they had shared on the bench that would be no more. Of course, no one had to spell out for Guidry that the bottom line was Berra's comfort and safety. The man *was* almost eighty-six years old, and there had been times in recent years when Guidry would glance over his shoulder to see Berra's chin drilling a hole in his chest.

As Guidry had once been mindful of the television camera to make sure Carmen didn't catch him slipping Yogi a tobacco stash, now he kept vigil for another reason. The last thing he was going to do was let the television audience get an up-close-and-personal look at Berra snoozing his way through the game.

As soon as the camera turned into the dugout, Guidry would stick an elbow into Berra's side and say, "Yogi, you see that?"

Startled awake, Berra would look around and say, "Naw, I missed it. What happened?"

"Oh, nothing," Guidry would say, potential embarrassment averted.

Guidry had considered it part of the deal, and he had loved every minute of it. But now it was over. It was time for the next phase and to be grateful for the time they'd had. "No matter how much I'd like to have him down there with me, he's better off up there now," Guidry reasoned. "It's better this way for his health."

And much better, he rationalized, than the inevitable alternative. "The important thing is that he's here," Guidry said, noting how Berra seemed more energized after a few days in Tampa than when he had arrived.

The move upstairs did provide one residual benefit for Guidry — a new round of ammunition in the endless game of good-natured teasing.

"Oh, you're too damn big to sit with us," he told Berra. "You're with the big brass now."

"Oh, yeah," Berra said with a smile.

But watching from his perch upstairs, the suite that once fit George Steinbrenner like a throne, Berra in a sense had actually replaced the Boss — in spirit if not in style — as the looming patriarch of the Yankees.

There were also concessions that Berra was stubbornly not ready to make. He had demonstrated as much a month before going to spring training when he insisted on flying to California to make his annual appearance at the Bob Hope Classic — even after organizers had failed to reach out to him, leaving Berra's family to assume that they were reluctant to host an unsteady eighty-five-year-old who could no longer play golf.

But Berra felt an obligation to attend, especially to Hope's wife, Dolores (who would pass away months later at the age of 102). As long as he could walk, why *wouldn't* he go? He could still handle the photo ops, schmooze with the players, and wave to the galleries. Nobody had the heart to tell him that the organizers had not requested his presence and might have decided to pursue younger celebrities.

A couple of weeks before the event, the Hope people were informed that Berra still wanted to come. In the end, no one objected. He went without incident, one last time.

Back at spring training, uniform or no uniform, Berra wasn't about to confine himself to the executive suite or to the city of Tampa, for that matter. One of the most pleasurable aspects of being in Florida was the opportunity to move around with the team, catch up with friends on the Grapefruit League circuit.

Berra didn't make all the trips. Some of the road games were a haul, a couple of hours at least when factoring in traffic. When Cucuzza, the clubhouse manager, would ask if he planned to make one of the longer drives, Berra would occasionally stick out his tongue, which meant no. Whenever possible, Berra preferred sign language to express displeasure or sentiment that was contrary.

As a manager, whenever he noticed his counterpart gesturing to him in disgust for a particular move, such as bringing in his closer early, Berra liked to put a thumb to his nose and wiggle his fingers, in nah-nah-nah-nah-nah fashion. Yogi being Yogi.

Fortunately, there were several teams within an hour's drive and people in those places Berra always looked forward to seeing when the opportunity presented itself. Kissimmee, where the Astros train, was one trip that Berra usually made, given his ties to the Houston organization dating back to his coaching days in the mid- to late 1980s. Besides the former owner, John McMullen, who died in 2005, Berra was close to Craig Biggio, the Astros star who retired in 2007 with 3,060 career hits. Biggio, out of Long Island, had come up as a catcher and credited Berra's mentoring for helping him to become an all-star behind the plate before making a shift to second base. Berra also made a point of checking in with Dennis Liborio, the team's longtime clubhouse manager.

Some of Berra's baseball relationships went back decades. Others he had developed in the years since his return to the Yankees, just by being around, being himself, dropping by opposing clubhouses to introduce himself to people he admired from afar or whose fathers he had known back in the day. Jim Leyland, who had idolized Berra as a child, was one manager Berra liked very much. Another was Boston's Terry Francona, who had always appreciated Berra reminiscing about his old man, Tito, in the 1950s.

One day at Yankee Stadium, Francona brought Berra into the Boston clubhouse, announcing, "Fellas, I just want to introduce you to the guy my dad says is the greatest clutch hitter he ever saw." Suddenly, Kevin Youkilis, David Ortiz, and the whole lot of them were giving the old Yankee a warm embrace, asking him to sign balls for them.

In early March 2011, Berra hit the road with the Yankees as they headed to Port Charlotte to play the Rays. He wanted to see Don Zimmer, now the Rays' senior adviser, and also Rays manager Joe Maddon, a fiftysomething hipster with whom Berra had formed a bond through Zimmer.

"What the hell are you listening to?" Berra had asked Maddon one day, settling in on the couch as the manager blasted Led Zeppelin. Berra, of course, had heard similar earsplitting music at home, having raised three boys of roughly the same age and musical generation as Maddon.

Maddon, born to an Italian father (whose name was shortened from Maddonini) and a Polish mother, grew up in the northeastern Pennsylvania town of Hazleton and liked to get Berra talking about the Hill in St. Louis. Berra, in turn, would query Maddon on his bold strategies — the defensive shift he used on the Yankees' Mark Teixeira, for instance — and especially liked to talk about the young Rays star Evan Longoria, who Berra had told a reporter reminded him of a young Joe DiMaggio.

"He's good-looking, dresses nice," Berra had said. "The girls go for him, too."

When this assessment was repeated to Longoria, he chuckled and said, "That's funny. He told me I reminded him of Mickey Mantle."

On the day Berra was getting an earful of Zeppelin, Longoria ambled into the office when he heard that Berra was there and bent over to give Yogi a hug. Noticing that Longoria's arms were heavily taped, Berra said, "You look like a mummy up there."

"Yogi, I'm hurting," Longoria said.

"Yeah, right," Berra said, who soon after presented Longoria with a ball to sign for his golf tournament. The request made Longoria blush.

When Berra accompanied the Yankees to Port Charlotte in March 2011, he went out to the field to see Maddon and Zimmer while the Rays were taking batting practice. Watching his guys hit, Maddon happened to turn his head as Berra approached and saw him catch his foot in an area of the grass covered by a small tarp. Berra stumbled forward, right into Maddon's embrace.

"Oh, my Lord, I see Yogi going down, falling, and I knew I had to do everything I could to catch him," Maddon said later, calling the catch his "best as a professional." No harm. No foul. No fuss.

The next night, Berra went out to dinner with Dave Kaplan, who was visiting from New Jersey with his college-age daughter and Stump Merrill. It was meatloaf night at Lee Roy Selmon's, where the waitresses greeted Berra with their usual fawning attention. He sat down and ordered a drink — exactly three ounces of Ketel One . . . in a glass with a specific number of ice cubes that shouldn't be too big . . . served between the salad and the main course.

But the waiter couldn't hear or understand what Berra was saying. While he was much too young to know the specifics, he realized from the fuss that was made over Berra when he entered the restaurant that he was a celebrity, and the young man quickly became embarrassed. "I'm . . . sorry," he stammered. "I didn't . . ."

Although on one level, the scene was comical, a *Seinfeld* skit, it was also uncomfortable, because Berra, for the moment, was unable to make himself clear. Finally, Merrill intervened, knowing exactly what Berra wanted. Happy to have the situation resolved, Berra spent the rest of the meal talking about the trips he was intending to make, especially the game coming up soon against the Phillies in Clearwater.

But Guidry wondered if going to Clearwater was a good idea. "I'm not making that trip, Yog," he said. "Got to stay behind and work with the young pitchers. Maybe you shouldn't go."

Whenever Berra traveled with the team, Guidry preferred to be around, especially now, after his promise to Carmen that he would look after Yogi. The drive was only twenty-five minutes, and Guidry knew the others would keep an eye on him. Still, Guidry felt person-ally responsible.

"Nah, it's no big deal," Berra said. "I have to go."

He insisted that there were several people in the Phillies organiza-tion he wanted to see, and he also was hoping to get a ball signed by Hall of Famer Mike Schmidt. Once Berra made up his mind, there was no talking him out of it. Guidry's father had the same quality. As much as he worried about Berra's safety, Guidry had to admire the man's resolve. He would not give in or give up.

On Thursday, March 10, Berra drove with Joe Girardi to the Phil-lies' ultramodern complex in Clearwater and relaxed inside the air-conditioned clubhouse while the Yankees waited around before going out to stretch and take batting practice. Noticing the buffet table in the middle of the room, Berra shuffled over to help himself to a cup of soup. Cup in hand, he took a sip and a step away from the table. In an instant, he was down.

From all around the room, there were shrieks and yelps. Gene Monahan was nearby, but with his back to Berra. He turned to see his old friend on the floor, on his behind. "Someone get the paramedics," the trainer yelled.

Nobody was immediately sure what had happened, why Berra had fallen, beyond the fact that he seemed to have landed, quite fortu-nately, on his butt. Standing nearby, Jorge Posada had watched the scene unfold, the cup of soup dropping along with Berra. "When he fell down, it sounded at first like he was joking," Posada said. "He said, 'The damn soup's too hot.'"

But Monahan, not having seen the fall, had no idea what had caused it. Had it been the soup? Had he caught his foot on the carpet? Had he, God forbid, had a seizure or stroke?

The one thing Monahan was certain of was that he was not tak-ing any chances with Guidry's valued package — and certainly not the man he considered to be "the kindest and most human individual I've ever met in the game."

In his forty-ninth year with the organization, and its head trainer since 1973, Monahan, who had survived throat cancer in 2009, was beginning what would be a celebrated last season on the job. He had been around long enough to judge how to react. "I've known Yogi for a very long time, and if I could have predicted one thing that would happen in that situation, it would have been that he didn't want to make a fuss," Monahan said.

Monahan saw right away when he knelt down over Berra that there was no blood, he was fully conscious, and he didn't appear to be having any kind of episode. He was dazed and of course embarrassed. Some of the soup had spilled onto his khaki pants.

The paramedics' office was adjacent to the clubhouse, and they arrived quickly to take Berra's pulse and blood pressure. Both were elevated, which might have been caused solely by the fright of the fall. Just the same, Monahan agreed with the paramedics that it was best to be cautious.

They decided to transport Berra to Morton Plant Hospital, a couple of miles away. But he became agitated when Monahan informed him of the plan. "I ain't doing that," he said. "I ain't going to no hospital. I'm OK. It was the soup."

But Monahan persisted, addressing Berra calmly and repeating that they just wanted to make sure he was all right. Still Berra resisted. Monahan repeated himself, calmly but firmly. Berra kept saying, "Carmen will worry." Watching close by, Joe Girardi felt goose bumps hearing Berra fret about his wife while he sat on the carpet. Monahan assured Berra that he wouldn't be at the hospital very long, just for a few tests, and that someone would call Carmen soon to let her know that it was all precautionary.

While an ambulance was summoned, one of the paramedics fetched a wheelchair. The Yankees immediately put the clubhouse in lockdown, making sure it was clear of media.

Sweeny Murti, on the beat for WFAN radio since 2001, or one year after Berra returned to spring training, was outside on the field when he heard there was some kind of commotion in the clubhouse.

Murti tried to walk through the dugout to the clubhouse but was told the area was off-limits. By the time he reached the main clubhouse entrance, the ambulance was pulling away — and word was spreading that Berra was inside.

"There apparently was an Associated Press reporter hanging around in the dugout, who heard that something had happened to Yogi," Murti said. "But nobody seemed to know exactly what."

It was Murti who had broken the news on WFAN that Berra had fallen outside his home the previous summer and would have to miss Old-Timers' Day. Now a chill swept over him when he found out it was Yogi who had been taken off so abruptly. Over the years, Murti and Berra had developed an easy rapport, chatting for a few minutes every day in Tampa — "my favorite part of spring training," Murti said — and whenever Berra appeared at the stadium during the season.

"You talk to players all year long, and a fair amount of the time you know they're not that interested," he said. "Here's one of the great legends of the game, and all he wants to do is spend a few minutes saying hello, talking about the game."

Murti would never forget Berra's sweet response in June 2009 when he bumped into him at the stadium the day after Mets second baseman Luis Castillo had dropped a routine pop-up with two outs in the ninth, gift-wrapping a victory for the Yankees over the Mets.

"What'd you think of the end last night, Yogi?" Murti asked.

Berra grabbed him by the arm and with a devilish twinkle in his eye said, "It ain't over 'til it's over."

Murti had that very thought when he heard they had rushed Berra to the hospital. He prayed it wasn't over. Then he went on the air to report the news — which was spreading fast and without some badly needed context.

Lindsay Berra was on the train from Montclair to Manhattan when the texts and e-mails began flooding her phone.

"Is your grandfather OK?"

"What happened to Yogi?"

"Oh, my God, I hope everything's all right."

She had no idea what any of her friends were talking about, but she guessed that something was up and it couldn't be good. She called her father, trying not to sound alarmed.

"Is Grandpa OK?"

"What do you mean?" Larry Berra said. "I just got off the phone with him a half-hour ago. He was fine."

But the word was out, crawling ominously across the CNN ticker: "Yankees great Yogi Berra taken to hospital after fall."

That set off a new round of calls. Larry phoned his mother, who happened to be en route to Tampa from West Palm Beach, where she had been visiting Jacqueline McMullen, the widow of John McMullen. Carmen told her son that she had already been contacted by the Yankees and that Yogi had slipped, was all right, and had been taken to the hospital just to be safe.

She soon reached Yogi — who at the time did not have a cell phone — on a hospital line. She knew he was fine because all he did was complain about having missed out on his chance to get his baseball signed by Mike Schmidt.

"It was just a little slip," Carmen Berra said. "But there was such a big commotion, all the news bulletins."

Back in Tampa, the news reached the Yankees' complex, stopping Guidry in his tracks. "Oh, shit," he said, already imagining what the hell he would tell Carmen. But first he needed more information. He didn't have Gene Monahan's cell phone number, so he called Steve Donohue, who assured him that Berra was not injured or ill and had probably lost his breath and balance when he tasted the hot soup.

Still, Guidry was worried. "Even that, you don't know," he said. "Donohue said that he fell on his behind — and we know he doesn't have a long way to go — but the man is [almost] eighty-six years old. Something could have been jarred by him just falling like that. You know how it is at that age — it's easy to break a bone, break your hip."

Until Berra was examined and released, Guidry was not going to

rest easy, though he took a moment to call Bonnie at home. He figured she would hear the news on television, and there was no point
in her becoming alarmed.

Berra reached the hospital shortly before noon. Donohue called
Guidry about ninety minutes later to say that the doctors had run
tests and that Berra had checked out fine. He would be released some-
time during the afternoon. Lou Cucuzza would pick him up and drive
him back to Tampa.

Having finished his work with the pitchers early, Guidry had left
the ballpark and was waiting at his apartment. Donohue told him that
Berra was already asking that Guidry meet him back at the park. *Only*
Guidry.

Not long after, his cell phone rang again. It was Cucuzza. "Someone wants to talk to you," he said. It was Berra, next to him in the car.

"Yogi, how're you feeling?" Guidry said.

"I'm OK," he said. "You at the park?"

"Yeah, I'm waiting for you right here."

"OK, don't leave."

Berra handed Cucuzza the phone, still agitated about having lost
the day, embarrassed by the fuss that had been made, and not at all
happy about having been administered medication by the doctor at
the hospital.

"He kept saying, 'The soup was too hot, that's all,'" Cucuzza said.
"And you know what? He was right. The soup in that clubhouse was
ridiculously hot. He was upset, but I think I was more upset just because he was. The guy's like your grandfather. He's everybody's grandfather."

Now Berra complained that Guidry had had his afternoon inter-
rupted. Cucuzza told him, "You know Gator doesn't mind." Berra
nodded. *By this point, how could he not know that?* Cucuzza thought.

"Everyone helps out with Yogi," he said. "But what Gator does,
year in and year out, that's on another level."

Twenty minutes later, Cucuzza pulled into the parking lot at the

Yankees' complex. Guidry was right where he said he'd be, leaning against his white Ford pickup. Berra got out of the car, muttering under his breath and moving with greater conviction, in Guidry's opinion, than he had all spring. He threw his bag into the back of the truck and continued to curse and complain all the way to the hotel.

"Yogi, they were just doing their jobs," Guidry said.

"Aw, I told them I was fine, didn't have any pain," he said. "It was the damn soup."

Guidry continued to harp on the need for caution, but Berra didn't want to hear it. As far as he was concerned, he had needlessly missed one of his favorite trips, another day of spring training. He hated wasting even a day.

But all was fine now. He was back in Tampa. He was with Guidry.

When they reached the hotel, Guidry made sure to walk Berra inside and up to his room. Carmen was there, waiting.

"You OK?" she said, giving him a hug.

"I'm fine, yeah," he said.

On some level, he at least knew the Yankees cared. In a couple of weeks, back in New York, they would take another opportunity to show him how much.

On the night of March 30, 2011, more than eleven hundred people jammed into a posh ballroom in a Sheraton hotel on the West Side of Manhattan for the Yankees' 32nd Welcome Home Dinner. It was a tradition begun under Steinbrenner and the only off-field event that every player was obligated to attend.

Fans and sponsors also were welcome, some plunking down about $15,000 for a table, with the proceeds going to the Yankees' charitable foundation.

The dinner had become a staple on Berra's calendar in 1999, when the Yankees celebrated his return by giving him the Pride of the Yankees award—which in 2011 was going to the retired pitcher Mike Mussina. In Yankee land, there is never any shortage of awards or recipients. In Berra's case, the organization had honored him every which way over a dozen redemptive years. This time it was the Yankees' Lifetime Achievement Award, which — truth be told — he had earned decades ago.

Five years earlier, Berra would have been appropriately proud but would probably have taken the night in stride. Now Steinbrenner was gone, and Berra was just a month and a half away from his eighty-sixth birthday. Emotions flowed more freely than ever.

The Berra family had a table. Larry, Dale, and Tim were there, along with granddaughter Lindsay and a few other family members. The table just happened to be near where JoAnna Garcia, Nick Swisher's wife, was sitting and taking every opportunity to tell any Berra whose attention she got that "Nick just loves Yogi." It would have been a challenge that night to find a single Yankee who didn't.

Berra knew he would have to make a speech, much as he hated doing so, and he'd asked Dave Kaplan to write a few words for him. Although he was dressed down — wearing a blue blazer, olive slacks, and his trusty Nicole Miller–designed baseball tie — he was nervous about having to stand up in front of the entire organization. Carmen, too, worried that he would be overcome by the occasion.

Suzyn Waldman, who was emceeing the dinner, was scheduled to introduce Berra. This was only fitting, as Waldman had, more than anyone with the possible exception of Steinbrenner, helped launch Berra's second life with the Yankees. She had been responsible for making this day "necessary" — to quote Berra's Hall of Fame induction speech. Before the dinner began, Carmen took a moment to whisper in Waldman's ear, "Make sure he doesn't lose it up there."

Waldman had grown close to the family — her Facebook profile photo for much of the 2011 season was one of her and Yogi, together in Tampa. "Don't worry," she told Carmen. "He'll be fine."

The Yankees had put together a short video tribute that included testimonials from Joe Girardi, Gene Monahan, and some of the players — Derek Jeter, Nick Swisher, Mariano Rivera. Berra watched from his seat at the family table as the old black-and-white clips of him more than half a century ago were interspersed with the testimonials in crystal-clear color.

How many technological changes had there been in the world since he had first put on the so-called tools of ignorance for the Yankees? How many wars had been fought since he had survived D-day? How many championship banners had the Yankees flown?

He was still here, ready for another Opening Day. But first Waldman had to call him to the dais. There was one more standing ovation as the players, seated at the surrounding tables, practically formed a protective wall around "the Greatest Living Yankee" as he moved slowly but steadily forward.

Reaching a glass podium emblazoned with the team's logo, Berra was presented the crystal award by Hal Steinbrenner, the Boss's younger son and now Yankees managing general partner. He stepped to the microphone and began by giving the audience what they wanted.

"Thank you for making this night necessary," he said to laughter and applause.

Then he turned serious, and the room grew silent, people straining to hear. "The Yankees," he said, "have always meant everything to me. They still do . . ."

He paused to dab his eyes. He tried to continue, but his voice began to crack.

Waldman, standing deliberately behind him, delivered on her promise to Carmen. She stepped forward and whispered in his ear, "If you cry, Yogi, there's no vodka tonight."

Berra smiled, regained his voice.

"Yankee fans are the best in the world," he said. "Here's to a great year. God bless."

Epilogue

Signing Off Till Spring

Ron Guidry finally made it to Cooperstown about fifteen hours late, according to Berra Standard Time, with the excuse that his flights from Louisiana through Atlanta had been delayed by storms. But here he was, bursting into the cramped backroom of TJ's Place, a restaurant on Main Street, and there was Berra, with a stack of *Sports Illustrated* magazines in front of him, pen in hand and a Yankees cap sitting high on his head.

Eyeing Goose Gossage stretched out in a chair to his right, Guidry picked right up where the fraternal clowning had left off the last time they had all been together, at Old-Timers' Day.

"Shit," he said to Gossage while pointing at Berra. "He won't sign for *me*. I got to pay the damn money."

Berra looked up from his tedious work and smiled. He was sitting behind a desk that was littered with baseball memorabilia, the area in front of him cleared so that he could put his autograph on a few dozen covers of the magazine that had featured him in its annual "Where Are They Now?" issue.

On this steamy late July weekend, Berra was exactly where he had been for years, save the previous one, 2010, when he had missed his beloved Hall of Fame induction weekend while recuperating in the hospital from the fall outside his home. One year later, it was no secret that the mishap had placed Berra at yet another fork in life's road. The cane propped against the side of the desk was evidence that in order to keep going, he needed some help.

The stumbles and soup spill in Florida were followed by another near fall at Joe Torre's charity golf tournament in Westchester County in June and a slip on a bathroom floor at an autograph show soon after. Kevin McLaughlin, the longtime family friend who considered himself Berra's protector at shows and gave himself the comic title of "senior signing consultant," grabbed him and turned white in the process.

"Goddamn it, Yogi, don't do that to me," he said.

"Aw, I'm fine, I'm fine," Berra said, still believing in the power of his protective bubble. "Don't worry."

His family and friends did worry, with good reason, but were also amazed and somewhat in awe of his determination to keep moving, not to let go of his baseball life. In Berra's mind, he had already missed one induction weekend too many. There was no way he wasn't going to Cooperstown and making his usual appearance at TJ's, where the legends of the game set up shop to sign for the masses.

"I think out of everything, including Old-Timers' Day, he loves this the most," McLaughlin said. "The Yankees are the Yankees, but he considers the Hall of Fame a special club."

Unlike Gossage, a 2008 inductee, it was a club that Guidry did not belong to, and the truth of the matter was that he didn't really need to be making the long trip back to New York so soon after Old-Timers' Day. Yes, he stood to make a few dollars for appearing at an autograph show or two, but nowhere near what Berra earned — anywhere from $20,000 to $50,000, depending on the location and size of the show.

Berra did only a few shows a year, and the money — though appreciated for what it could do for his grandchildren — was no longer the motivation. The people closest to him would swear on a stack of old Yankees yearbooks that it never had been.

"He loves being out there, being Yogi and around these guys," McLaughlin said. "You can't get him to stop."

Guidry put it differently, more emphatically. "He has to keep going, or he's going to shut down," he said.

Therein was the reason for Guidry's presence in Cooperstown — though only at gunpoint would he ever have admitted that he was there mainly because it made Berra happy. Eleven years after their first spring training together in Tampa, Berra counted on Guidry to walk into the backroom at TJ's and stir up shit the way he always did.

When Ted Hargrove, the owner of the restaurant, told Guidry that he looked tanned and toned — as he always did — Hargrove assumed that Guidry must have spent a lot of time on the golf course during spring training. "Hell, no," Guidry said. "Goose, here, he was playing all the time. Me, I was too busy taking care of this guy."

He pointed again at Berra and said, "That's my job, my very full-time job."

"Hardest damn job you ever had," Gossage said, playing along.

Having gotten in his jabs, Guidry walked over to Berra to pay his respects.

"How you feeling, Yog?" he said, leaning over to share a hushed conversation until Gossage intervened by asking, "Gator, how come you couldn't get out of Atlanta?"

"I don't know," Guidry said. "Maybe they didn't want my ass to take away the attention from this son of a bitch right here."

With a fresh stack of magazines in front of him, Berra resumed signing, firmly and meticulously, nothing like the standard celebrity scribble. He took his cue on that from the men he considered the masters of legibility, Ted Williams and Joe DiMaggio.

"They had beautiful signatures," Berra said in a reverent tone. He bristled over how modern players' signatures tended to be indistinguishable. For clarity's sake, whenever Berra asked one of the kids like Evan Longoria to sign a ball, he would also request that they write their number under the name.

While Berra signed, Guidry and Gossage began telling old war stories, hoping there was someone in the room who hadn't heard them before. If not, well, too bad, the memories got better with age and occasionally a little more dramatic as well.

Somehow they got on the subject of the late-seventies Yankees' futility at the old Seattle Kingdome, where the Mariners didn't seem capable of beating anyone but them. Guidry remembered pitching there one night during the 1979 season and being undone by perhaps the strangest play he'd ever seen.

"Something crazy always happened in that place, but this one, un-*freaking*-believable," he said.

He was standing in the middle of the room, recounting how he had taken a one-run lead into the ninth inning, when he'd loaded the bases with two outs and Leon Roberts, an average right-handed hitter with decent home run power, coming to the plate.

"So I throw him a good slider in on the hands, and he pops it up down the first-base line, way the hell up there," he said, pantomiming a windup, clucking his tongue for the crack of the bat, and doing a little dance to demonstrate how Chris Chambliss had circled under the ball in foul territory.

"So what happens?" Guidry continued. "The ball hits one of those damn speakers and comes down in fair territory between first base and home. I'm right here. Chambliss is there. Willie Randolph is coming in from second. We're standing there, and, *boop,* the ball bounces off the hard turf right between us with a crazy spin and back into foul territory before anyone can pick it up. Foul ball!"

Guidry shook his head and said, "And what happens next?"

He wound up again and clucked again, only louder this time.

"Home run — grand slam — and we lose another damn game in the dome."

He turned and pointed at Berra, whose rapt attention he already had.

"You were there, right, Yog?" Guidry said.

Berra nodded, dutifully.

"Yeah," Gossage said, "but you wouldn't let me come into the game, would you?"

Guidry waved him off. "*Sheeet,*" he said, stretching out the word with his Cajun lilt. "I'll lose the damn game by myself."

(Let the record show that Guidry did lose to the Mariners on July 10, 1979, when Leon Roberts homered after his pop fly struck a speaker 150 feet high, rolled over the top of it, and fell harmlessly into foul territory. But it happened early in the game. Guidry went only six innings that night, and George Steinbrenner was so incensed about losing again to the Mariners that he ordered an extra workout for the team. Bucky Dent was the only regular to show up.)

Stories told, misremembered or embellished, it was time for Berra, Guidry, and Gossage to go outside. It was almost high noon. The line of autograph seekers for Berra already stretched down the block.

There were two tables set up, one on each side of the front entrance to the restaurant. Berra and Guidry were situated at the one to the left. Gossage joined his fellow Hall of Fame reliever Rollie Fingers and the great San Francisco Giants pitcher Juan Marichal to the right.

For the next hour, there were at least five people in line to see Berra for every one person en route to the Gossage-Fingers-Marichal table. The fans brought photos, bats, balls, caps, gloves, and the occasional piece of clothing to be signed at prices that varied based on the item. Many came just to lean across the table, press a shoulder to Berra's, and have a photo snapped. Fathers pushed their young sons forward and told them not to be afraid to shake the grandfatherly legend's hand.

While signing sporadically — there were no two-for-one deals — Guidry provided an ongoing color analysis. He told one female fan not to be fooled by Berra's age and recounted the Tampa shopping story, when Berra had insisted that they trail an attractive young woman up and down the aisles.

Another woman said, fawning, "He's so cute."

A woman even older than Berra, age eighty-eight, came with her granddaughter to have him sign her beautiful white sweater with a Sharpie. (Berra was reluctant to ruin the sweater and talked her into a more conventional autograph.)

A middle-age man thanked him "for coming out and doing stuff like this."

Yes, he was being well compensated, but could the fans imagine their own octogenarian parents or grandparents sitting patiently for an hour in such oppressive heat, shaking hand after sweaty hand, smiling in every pose — which he prided himself on doing?

The fiftyish Kevin McLaughlin couldn't. "I go with him to these things, and I'm tired afterward," he said. "I don't know how he does it."

Not so easily anymore, in fact, and that became obvious to Guidry after about an hour of signing. He could see that Berra was fading in the afternoon steam bath. The line of fans remained long, but a cool drink inside along with a rest — or a nap — seemed like a good idea.

Guidry whispered to Berra and then took it upon himself to call a time-out. He helped Yogi up — chagrined by how Berra struggled to stand after sitting so long — and they went inside. On the way to the back, Berra insisted on stopping at a table to say hello to Pete Rose, the banned all-time hits leader, who struck an isolated and lonely pose when appearing in Cooperstown to peddle his tainted name.

In many ways, Berra was the anti-Rose, welcome in every clubhouse in any ballpark. "The most loved man in America," Guidry said, before predicting — correctly, as it turned out — that the line outside TJ's would re-form as soon as Berra was ready to return.

On the day after the autograph show, Berra, Guidry, and a couple of other players went to the Otesaga, the historic Cooperstown hotel and resort, to meet a disabled boy at the request of Ted Hargrove. About the time they were ready to leave, a group of players' wives — Carmen Berra included — were finishing a luncheon there and were exiting the hotel to board a bus for an afternoon outing.

Guidry was sitting in a car, waiting for Berra, who was busy greeting all the wives as they exited the hotel, and Gossage, who had his back turned to Guidry while talking to Juan Marichal and one or two other players.

"Where's Yogi?" Guidry asked Kevin McLaughlin, saying he wanted to get going.

"He's over in the front with all the wives," McLaughlin said.

Guidry decided it was time to get Berra's attention and have some fun in the process. He got out of the car and yelled at the top of his lungs. *"Hey, come on, you dirty old man!"*

To which Gossage — in a classic "Who, me?" moment — turned around.

"Not *you*," Guidry said. "*That* dirty old man." He pointed at Berra, whose face lit up with a smile.

What cracked up McLaughlin — besides Gossage assuming that *he* was the dirty old man — was that Berra, the American icon, paid no mind to being called that in a crowded public place in which people had no way of knowing the nature of his relationship with Guidry. "But that's the way it is with Yogi if you're one of his real friends," McLaughlin said. "He doesn't want to be treated like a superstar or a celebrity. He wants his friends to bust his balls. He loves it. And nobody does it better than Gator."

But then, McLaughlin added, there was the serious point in the weekend, when it was time for them to part. "That's when you really see the love," he said.

In 2011, the goodbyes actually unfolded in stages — the first one coming in spring training, when Guidry delivered Berra to the Tampa Airport, where he would be met at the curb by an airport employee and helped through security and on to the gate.

"When we get there, I mean, I can't walk in, so it has to be quick," Guidry said. "We get out of the truck, and I ask him if he has everything. But we're both sad because, you know, that's it, the time together has ended again. One minute I was looking forward to picking him up, then it's three or four weeks later, and before you know it, it's over. It goes so fast, and for me it's like, *Oh, God, I hate this part.* When I go to hug him, it's this lonesome feeling."

Of course, Guidry knew they would see each other again within a couple of months, but the emptiness came with the recognition that spring training was their special shared adventure, their forever sleepaway camp, their club of two.

"It's so special to me because, I guess, of the trust he has in me," Guidry said. "Whether you want to call it love on his part for letting me do what I do with him all the time, I don't know. I can't say. But for me, to spend the time that I do is my way of showing the respect I have for him. It's not a burden. It's something I look forward to.

"I guess in a small way, all the little things he helped me accumulate when I was a player, maybe in some way I'm repaying the kindness, and sometimes I feel what I'm doing might even not be good enough. I don't expect that he thinks I owe him anything, but I've always felt that that's the way I should carry myself in the Yankee tradition. He's one of the last surviving members of those great Yankee times, an idol to millions. When you go all over with him and you watch the way people react, that's only fortifying what you already know."

From the time Guidry was let go by the Yankees as pitching coach, it occurred to him that Berra might also be *his* last hold on the game that he loved, and whenever Berra stopped going to spring training, that might be it for him, too.

Emotionally, it had come to the point where he was more prepared to give up the Yankees than he was to lose Berra. "I don't feel like I owe anything to the Yankees or that they owe anything to me," he said. "I'll go as long as Yogi goes, that's for sure. I didn't know the relationship would bloom into this. That's not why I did what I did. I just did it because I love the old man. You can't help but love him. I say it over and over — he's my best friend, and the game of baseball brought us together."

In Cooperstown, they shared some laughs, did their shows, went out to dinner, and watched Bert Blyleven and Roberto Alomar get inducted into the Hall of Fame. Then it was time to really say goodbye.

Time for Guidry to return to Louisiana, where he would recount the weekend to Bonnie, catch her up on the inside scoops, admit how upsetting it had been to see Berra struggle to get up and walk, how the reality of his age had finally hit home. But Guidry also would begin to anticipate and look forward to the first frog legs call from New Jersey.

For Berra's part, he would return to Montclair and keep trying to move forward as fast as he could. He would go to the stadium for the first game of every series and would suffer with the Yankees when they lost at home to Jim Leyland's Tigers in the heartbreaking fifth game of the American League Division Series. He would leave the ballpark that night mumbling under his breath about how the Yankees had failed to hit in the clutch.

"Wait till I see Swish in spring training," he would say, already plotting another tutorial with Nick Swisher, a playoff washout, assuming he would be back in New York. "Damn, he was trying to pull everything against the Tigers, trying to crush it. Don't know why he wasn't going with the pitch like he used to." Or as Berra had advised him to in the dugout on that glorious Tampa afternoon during spring training 2010.

One day, as the leaves turned yellow around Montclair, he would even feel spry enough to drop a bombshell on Dave Kaplan and some of the folks at the museum: he was going to try to convince Carmen to let him drive again, if only in the daytime — a motion he conceded she was not likely to second. (If anything, Carmen would consider live-in help as Yogi continued to take the occasional spill.)

Everyone around him nodded and thought: *What is with this man? What in the world is driving Mr. Yogi?*

But before any of that could happen, before Berra would get into the limousine with Carmen and Kevin McLaughlin for the long, scenic drive from Cooperstown to Montclair and Guidry would get into another limo heading to the city, they had to say goodbye. Until next year, next season, until it was time for the pitcher and catcher to meet again, the way it happened every spring.

And in that moment, Guidry could admit to harboring a deep-seated fear of the future and to not wanting his best friend to see his eyes moisten. He could admit to saying a silent prayer that Berra would indeed be back and that he would in fact see him again.

"Look, we all know that at some point in time, it's going to end," Guidry said. "He's going to stop going to Florida. This can't be forever."

But spring training always did symbolize hope, the power of renewal, one more chance. So Guidry embraced Berra and spoke to him in the tone that Berra loved best, the one guaranteed to make him smile.

"I'll see your ass in Tampa next year, OK?"

Berra did smile and surrendered to the hug.

"OK, kid," he said, nodding. "See ya then."

Postscript

On Old-Timers' Day, 2012, Yogi Berra struggled with what had long been a simple choice of ceremonial attire. What would be the most suitable match for his famed number eight Yankees' jersey?

Full uniform dress was out, that much was certain, and had been since Berra had broken the news to Ron Guidry the previous year at spring training: he no longer was up to the challenge of on-field activity. He realized there would be a small number of ex-Yankees as old or older than him — Bobby Brown and Jerry Coleman, to name two — who would be decked out in complete pinstriped regalia. And while it was painful for him to even think of being unable to join them and all the relative young'uns — most of all, Guidry — Berra had more pressing issues than how he looked, the worst of which was that he could hardly walk.

At eighty-seven, circulatory problems in his legs and feet required him to use a cane on his best days, a walker or wheelchair on his worst. Getting around had become such a chore that Berra — having spent only a few days at spring training in the vigilant and constant company of Guidry and others — had in a span of a few trying weeks moved into an assisted-living facility and practically withdrawn from public life. But not quite: there was still the matter of occasions he couldn't bring himself to miss.

He had already celebrated his birthday, May 12, at Yankee Stadium, where he arrived to find Guidry — "Driving Mr. Yogi" cap sitting atop his combed-back hair — waiting behind the outfield fence alongside a golf cart. Guidry's attendance had been a closely guarded secret, and Berra's face lit up when he spotted his old friend, who proceeded to drive him around the dirt track, all the way to home plate. There, a cake awaited them, along with a prolonged and heartfelt ovation.

On the day his annual golf tournament was rained out in early June, most of the invited guests made the drive to the Montclair Golf Club. A sedentary Berra, propped against a pillow in a large leather chair to ease the pain in his back, greeted them like an ailing head of state. When the rescheduled tournament date came around in July, he returned to the club on a bright sunny day and surprised everyone by lasting into the dinner hour. His effort proved well worth it.

When the hired entertainment — a cast member from the hit show *Jersey Boys* — got up to sing "Oh, What a Night," Guidry, who didn't have to be asked twice to fly in from Louisiana for the event, bounded to the front and pulled Mickey Rivers and Willie Randolph up with him. Yogi and Carmen beamed like proud and tickled parents while the three Yankees mainstays from two seventies championship teams staged their own abbreviated comic version of *Dancing with the Stars*.

On the third weekend of July, Berra would even confound his doctors and loved ones by insisting on making the long drive to Cooperstown for the Hall of Fame induction weekend, despite Guidry being unable to join him.

But the gaps between celebratory occasions were long and languorous for Berra, who had abandoned his custom of attending the opening game of every home series at the stadium. To make this difficult period much, much worse, Carmen had fallen ill and required a recuperative hospital stay. This led the Berra sons to the logical but painful conclusion that their parents were no longer safe in their

Montclair colonial, with its spiral staircase and other features potentially hazardous to the elderly. A family decision was made to move them into an assisted-living facility in a nearby town.

That also meant, at least for a while, that Yogi would have to stay in the rehabilitation wing before moving into the new apartment. His mind remained sharp, his upper body strong, and therapists believed they could strengthen his legs and help him move about with less discomfort. But Berra, the Greatest Living Yankee, suddenly found himself living and eating among the neediest residents, the failing and the infirm.

For the most part, he kept to himself throughout the rehab process, but one night he did have a surprise visitor. A woman named Irene, clearly disoriented, burst into his room and began to undress. Berra rang for help and later seemed more amused than upset by the incident. He told a less-intrusive visitor, "She didn't go too crazy."

It was at the facility where his trusted museum staff members, Dave Kapan and Joni Bronander, picked him up on the Sunday morning of the Yankees' sixty-sixth Old-Timers' Day, on the first of July. They could tell he was nervous, even if he wouldn't admit it, worrying about his stamina, fussing over his pants. Should he go with the light-colored pair that would be more comfortable? Or a darker shade that would better hide any perspiration or, God forbid, a stain if his bladder should happen to betray him? Men considerably younger than Berra had to wrestle with such issues. Considering the circumstances, it was understandable that this man of energy and action was finally feeling his age.

He ultimately chose the lighter tan slacks to go with his museum polo shirt, and off they went to Yankee Stadium, where Debbie Tymon, the Yankees' senior vice president of marketing, had meticulously planned Berra's day from the moment he arrived. A golf cart waited for him in the parking deck. Joe Flannino of stadium operations greeted him with a wheelchair and an EMS worker, and both were ordered to accompany the legend wherever he went.

"We knew it wasn't certain that Yogi would be coming," Tymon said. "But I told Dave, 'If he's able to make it I guarantee that we'll make it as easy for him as possible. He will experience the day with dignity.'"

She had already dealt with the far more daunting challenge of having a grand and proud Yankee elder make a rare public appearance under less-than-ideal conditions. In 2008, seventy-eight-year-old George Steinbrenner attended the All Star Game at the old Yankee Stadium during its final season, before the move to the palatial new ballpark across the street. The Boss, two years prior to his death, was in no condition to walk or even stand. After a rousing introduction of forty-nine Hall of Fame players at their respective positions, later joined by the starting lineups of the American and National Leagues, Steinbrenner was delivered by cart, along with a few specially marked baseballs to be used for a series of "first pitches" by selected Yankees greats.

Berra was one of them, of course, and he cherished the moment, but would also recall it with a lingering sadness over how much a weeping Steinbrenner had physically declined.

Tymon had big plans for Berra on Old-Timers' Day, too, but that was for later. Upon arrival, Berra only wanted to "see the guys." From the parking deck he was wheeled into the bowels of the ballpark, headed to the makeshift old timers' clubhouse. The room was closed to reporters, who gathered outside. As Berra approached for his first public exposure in his newly and quite apparent disabled state, the reporters were more than startled. They were subdued. Who among the hardened media didn't have an enduring love or at least a genuine soft spot for Lawrence Peter Berra?

Seemingly on cue, Guidry appeared at the entrance as a one-man welcoming committee. "Hey, buddy, you made it," he said, reaching over to gently squeeze Berra's shoulders. They went inside, where Berra's wheelchair was stationed in the center of the room and was immediately surrounded. Mel Stottlemyre pulled up a seat, as did Bobby Richardson, followed by Bobby Brown, who happened to have been Berra's first major league roommate. Ralph Terry—who threw the ninth-inning pitch to Bill Mazeroski that sailed over Berra's head in left field and out of Pittsburgh's Forbes Field to end the 1961 World Series—asked to have his cap autographed. Darryl Strawberry placed a ball and pen in Berra's hand.

When Berra spotted his beloved battery mate, Whitey Ford, eighty-four, he summoned his strongest voice and said, "Whitey's almost as old as me."

Ford, dealing with some memory loss, hadn't forgotten that. "Yeah," he said. "Yogi's one hundred, I'm ninety."

Seeing his old pal Stump Merrill, the organization lifer who had never been invited to an old-timers' event, Berra needled, "What took you so long?"

"Yog, what can I say?" Merrill said. "It only took me thirty-six years." Merrill was delighted to see how much Berra was amused by his self-deprecation. He could also admit that he wished he'd come sooner, considering the sobering sight of Berra—with whom he had shared all those walks along spring training outfield warning tracks—stuck in a wheelchair.

"It's tough to watch, to be honest," he said. "I mean, I love the man. He brought me to the big leagues and I'm indebted to him in so many ways. I've stayed close to him. All I can tell you is when the day comes that he isn't here at all, it'll be a sad, sad day for a lot of people."

Seized with emotion by the mere thought, Merrill coughed and pursed his lips.

"No question, he's sensitive about people seeing him in the chair," he continued, his voice softer now. "He's a proud man. He told me, 'Stump, I'm getting therapy. I'm getting better.' It kills him to not be able to put the whole uniform on, but the one thing I knew was that he would be here today no matter how he had to come—in a wheelchair, carried in, or whatever—because this is all he knows. And I don't mean it the way it necessarily sounds—this is a man who loves the people in his life. But if we were in assisted living, we'd all be depressed and would need something like this to put us back in touch with who we are. Being here, surrounded by all these guys, this is who Yogi is and that's one of the reasons why he's such a great man."

Watching the frivolity from the side, Guidry took measure of the greatness in all its late-in-life glory, taking a mental snapshot of the look on Berra's face. "He's in his element, he lives for this," Guidry said. "And I guarantee you in a few minutes he'll want to be wheeled all the way down to the other end of the goddamned stadium to go see the guys over there, too."

He meant the contemporary players, especially his favorites, like Derek Jeter and Nick Swisher. Guidry knew Berra like the back of his pitching hand. When the old timers drifted in small groups out onto the field for batting practice and interviews, Berra had Flannino wheel him down the corridor and into the Yankees clubhouse. Swisher — again the only active player to have attended Berra's golf tournament — was the first to rush over. Then Jeter came, followed by a host of others. As a bonus, Mariano Rivera — injured and out for the season — happened to be in the house. Ready with a greeting that was perfect for the occasion, Berra addressed the forty-two-year-old Rivera as "old-timer." Rivera smiled and kissed him on the top of his Yankees cap.

Finally it was time for the festivities, for the introduction of the old-timers, for Debbie Tymon's carefully planned program to begin.

"Making sure Yogi was comfortable was the most important thing but not the only thing," she said. "I mean, with Mr. Steinbrenner it was different. He was the Boss, the only owner. Yogi was one of sixty-six old-timers and even if he was the most famous, we didn't want to single him out as the only one who couldn't walk or run out of the dugout."

Having already had Guidry drive Berra in from the outfield on his birthday, Tymon had another brilliant stroke of ceremonial choreography: Berra and the five old-timers who were Hall of Fame members would get the golf cart treatment after the introduction of the others massed in the dugout. They would come in pairs: first Rickey

Henderson riding with Jerry Coleman, the former Yankees' second baseman who had made the Hall as a broadcaster; then Goose Gossage and Reggie Jackson; and finally Berra alongside Ford, the teammate he'd asked for, driven by Flannino.

Before taking the ride in from the outfield, Berra was helped on with his jersey. He asked if it was all right to not tuck it into his pants, to let it hang over his belt. Of course, he was told. Wear it out. Wear it any way you like. Ford, retired number sixteen, told him to stop being a pain in the ass. They laughed and then basked in the cheers of the crowd on the way to join the others. But the mood turned solemn during the annual scrolling of names from the Yankees' family, lost since the previous summer.

Once Berra had joked — unwittingly, of course — that he hoped he would never see his name "up there." But the years now seemed to have gone by in a blur. The most important losses — the boys of summer themselves — continued to mount. Bill "Moose" Skowron's name flashed on the screen; the death of the former first baseman — a treasured teammate and friend — had really hurt.

With the introductions completed, the old-timers began stretching in preparation for their casual two-inning affair that promised to be a sticky challenge on what had turned into a brutally hot afternoon. Several gathered round the cart to give Berra a handshake or hug. Guidry waited his turn before stepping up to say goodbye and that they would speak to each other soon.

It had been many years since Berra had participated in the exhibition of geezers, but he would typically hang around the dugout, poking fun, inhaling the atmosphere. Not today, though. Fatigued by the excitement and the exertion, he was more than ready to leave. Flannino steered the cart around the track, through the outfield gate, and within minutes Berra was back in the car, heading up the Deegan Expressway to the George Washington Bridge.

He was quiet on the forty-five minute ride home, no doubt relieved the appearance was over and had gone off without a hitch. He was looking forward to relaxing in his room for the rest of the day, conserving his strength for the physical therapy that would resume in the next day or two.

In the ensuing weeks, Berra would approach his rehab no differently than any other task he had taken on in his storied life. Hard work was all the man ever knew. Eventually his condition improved to where he began walking more steadily with a cane, if only for short distances. In September, he attended an event at the museum with Don Larsen, who was generating publicity for the auctioning of his perfect game jersey to raise money for his grandchildren's educations. Yogi and Carmen were again spotted in their favorite Montclair restaurants, out for an early bird dinner. One September day, as the Yankees struggled to hold off the charging Baltimore Orioles in the race for the division crown, Berra even telephoned Kaplan and asked to be driven to the stadium for a game, hours before a single fan would settle into a seat.

There was legitimate hope that he was rallying, giving living, breathing testimony of the Yankees' famed five o'clock lightning. He was even calling Guidry again, nagging him about frog legs and other assorted subjects, but mostly about hooking up during the 2013 spring training. But October and the postseason at Yankee Stadium came and went without an appearance by Berra, which only emphasized the uncertainty of his situation and the need for him to take life easy, one day at a time.

If all of his plans had to be classified as questionable, that was still an improvement on the prognosis that would have been made on Old-Timers' Day, when the mere notion of ever meeting up with Guidry again for good times in Tampa seemed impossible. The morbid view was that he might even have been saying goodbye.

After the car arrived at his new home that sultry afternoon, Berra moved slowly through the lobby, making his way past residents in wheelchairs, most of them women who were silent, whose heads were down and who did not react to the man still wearing his cap and jersey, holding tight to his walker.

A few of the facility's attendants, however — women with Caribbean accents — cheerfully told him that they had seen him on TV and that he'd looked great.

"Thanks," Berra said, smiling weakly, wanting only to get to his room, where he settled on the bed and asked Joni Bronander to turn on the television while he made himself comfortable to watch the Yankees play the White Sox. Staring back at Berra from the opposite side of the room, from the top of a chest of drawers, were two framed photos. One was of Carmen, holding their new great-grandchild. The other was of Yogi alongside Ron Guidry, with Guidry's arm around Berra's shoulder. The accompanying caption summarized the poignant reunion of a pitcher and a catcher that happened every spring for the past dozen years:

"Best Buddies: Gator and Mr. Yogi."

Acknowledgments

I first wrote about the relationship between Yogi Berra and Ron Guidry for the *New York Times* during spring training 2011. Interviewing Guidry outside the Yankees' clubhouse in Tampa, listening to him talk about his love for "the old man," brought tears to my eyes. I knew I had stumbled onto something quite rare and guessed — correctly, as it turned out — that there was much more to the story than a 1,500-word newspaper article could convey.

To my editors at the *Times* — Joe Sexton, Sandy Keenan, and Jay Schreiber — thank you for being so kind to the story and pushing to land it on A-1. My agent, Andrew Blauner, picked up the ball from there and encouraged me to pursue the project. Soon after, we were incredibly fortunate when Susan Canavan of Houghton Mifflin Harcourt burst into the room with her extraordinary energy and passion for envisioning, shaping, and editing the book. Thank you, Ashley Gilliam, for keeping us connected and focused, and Barbara Jatkola and Beth Burleigh Fuller for your deft handling of the manuscript.

Without Dave Kaplan's help on all things Yogi, this would have been a much more formidable task. Thank you to Ron and Bonnie Guidry for opening their home and their hearts. To Carmen and Yogi, my Montclair neighbors, I can only say bravo, you enrich our community and the country. Thank you to the Berra brothers — Larry, Tim, and Dale — and a special nod to granddaughter Lindsay for sharing her insights, along with her crispy bacon at the Bluestone.

Books are hard. They require an early morning discipline I never had as a young man and the encouragement and support of many people. They snatch away huge chunks of life. Fortunately, I had Alex Araton, my quick-fingered son, to transcribe interviews (with some of his beloved Yankees), along with the budding sports journalist Emily Kaplan. I had my amazing wife, Beth Albert, to read back and tolerate my ramblings, and my son Charly Araton to keep me entertained during our lunchtime breaks.

Thanks, as always, to my family and friends, who help keep me quasi-sane: my mother, Marilyn Araton, and her significant other, Abe Babitzky; my aunt Ruth Finkelstein; my in-laws, David and Ruth Albert; my sisters, Sharon Kushner and Randi Waldman; my nieces, Mindy Kushner-Hall, Devon Albert-Stone, and Emma Albert-Stone; my nephews, David Kushner, Matt Waldman, and LeJuan Hall; my sisters-in-law, Dana Albert and Hilary Albert; my brothers-in-law, Ashley Stone and Allan Waldman. To my special cousins, Stan and Richie Finkelstein and Gail Kashubo — our fathers would have appreciated this one.

Harvey Araton
Montclair, New Jersey

Index